Critical Perspectives
on Mental Health

O   o
cr   d
fr   o
ex   h
id   e
pe
                                               k
cr   l
de   y
of   c
th   s
–   e
au   y
of   l
cr   s
wl   t
ce

Vi   ,
E   s
at

Critical Perspectives on Mental Health

Vicki Coppock and John Hopton

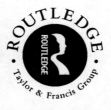

London and New York

First published 2000
by Routledge
11 New Fetter Lane, London EC4P 4EE

Simultaneously published in the USA and Canada
by Routledge
29 West 35th Street, New York, NY 10001

Transferred to Digital Printing 2004

Routledge is an imprint of the Taylor & Francis Group

© 2000 Vicki Coppock and John Hopton

Typeset in Times by Taylor & Francis Books Ltd
Printed and bound in Great Britain by
Selwood Printing Ltd, West Sussex

British Library Cataloguing in Publication Data
A catalogue record for this book is available from the British Library

Library of Congress Cataloging in Publication Data
Coppock, Vicki.
    Critical Perspectives on Mental Health / Vicki Coppock and
John Hopton.
    Includes bibliographical references and index.
    1. Psychiatry – philosophy – case studies. 2. Antipsychiatry –
case studies. I. Hopton, John, 1956– . II. Title.
    RC437.5 .C67   2000
    616.89'001–dc21   99-046626

ISBN 1–857–28879–3 (hbk)
ISBN 1–857–28880–7 (pbk)

Contents

Acknowledgements

As each of us has written different chapters and has therefore had different kinds of help from different people, it seems appropriate for us each to write our own acknowledgements before acknowledging those people who assisted us both.

Vicki Coppock would like to thank Paul Reynolds for his ongoing interest in this work and his valuable comments in relation to Chapters 1, 2, 5 and 6. Sincere thanks also go to the many friends and colleagues who have 'been there' over the last couple of years, giving so much time, understanding and support when times were hard – you know who you are!! Finally, enduring love and thanks go to Johnathan and Andrew Coppock whose love and patience knows no bounds and makes it all worthwhile.

John Hopton wishes to thank Joe Berke, Michael Conran, John Heaton, Juliet Mitchell, Leon Redler and Stephen Ticktin, for answering questions about David Cooper, R. D. Laing and the early days of the Philadelphia Association. Although they may not realize it, conversations with David Clark, Craig Fees, David Glenister, George Hoggarth and Sue White were important in helping John clarify his own thoughts about mental health, mental distress and mental health care. Sue Hopton, Siân Hopton and Aidan Hopton have been very patient and understanding during the two and a half years it has taken to complete this book.

Together we would like to thank Kathryn Chadwick and Phil Scraton for their hard work in establishing and sustaining the Centre for Studies in Crime and Social Justice (CSCSJ) at Edge Hill College of Higher Education, Ormskirk, Lancashire. Their enthusiasm for and commitment to social justice has confirmed 'the Centre' as a stimulating and supportive environment for the development of critical research and writing. The content of this book largely reflects the principles and priorities of our teaching and research within the CSCSJ. Many other colleagues in the CSCSJ have given us support and encouragement from the conception through to the completion of this book and we are most grateful to them. Finally, special thanks go to Barbara Houghton for her invaluable advice on preparing the final manuscript.

Vicki Coppock and John Hopton
June 1999

Introduction

Since the late 1950s, one of the most striking features of the published literature on mental health is the plethora of books and articles which challenge the assumptions of mainstream medical psychiatry and clinical psychology. Two of the best known generalized critiques of psychiatry are those associated with Thomas Szasz and Ronald David Laing (see Clare, 1976). However, there are other perspectives which are at least equally significant. These include: Michel Foucault's influential, but historically inaccurate, account of the confinement of mentally distressed people and the emergence of medical psychiatry; the labelling theory perspective associated with Thomas Scheff; later work by former colleagues of Laing and others associated with the Philadelphia and Arbours Associations; anti-racist psychiatry; feminist critiques of psychiatry; the radical anti-therapy perspectives associated with Peter Breggin and Jeffrey Masson; and autobiographical accounts of mental health services by users and ex-users of those services. One theme common to these perspectives is that to varying degrees and in a variety of different ways they all take issue with theoretical perspectives associated with medical psychiatry and/or mainstream clinical psychology and with the socio-legal power which psychiatrists have in many countries of the world.

However, despite the existence of this broad spectrum of critical material, there has been relatively little literature bringing these critiques together in any cohesive way. Nor is it openly acknowledged that many of the so-called critical perspectives resonate with the ideas of liberal reformers *within* mainstream psychiatry. Notable exceptions are Lucy Johnstone's *Users and Abusers of Psychiatry* (1989) and Ian Parker *et al.*'s *Deconstructing Psychopathology* (1995). Yet these books stop short of synthesizing disparate critiques into a comprehensive critical theory of mental health, or of explaining the relationship between such radical standpoints and other mainstream ideas about human psychology and mental health. Furthermore, while self-styled critics of psychiatry criticize psychiatry and clinical psychology for interpreting ambiguous research findings to support prevailing ideological assumptions, some of them are equally inclined to ignore research which challenges their own perspectives. For example, while |Thomas Szasz's work makes a valuable contribution to our understanding of the *precipitating* factors in the causation of mental distress, he has shown a marked reluctance to consider seriously the possibility that there may be biological factors |which *predispose* people to certain forms of mental distress. Taken to its logical conclusion, such reluctance could result in failure to invest in psychopharmacological research such as that which has led to the development of a drug such as Prozac (fluoxetine). While the use of psychoactive medications remains controversial, there is evidence that some doctors and some users of mental health services have more positive attitudes towards newer psychoactive drugs such as Prozac, than they do to some older products (see Calabrese and Markovitz, 1991; Greenberg *et al.*, 1994). This is not to say that such new drugs are flawless, but it does suggest a need for more research into both psychopharmacology and consumer satisfaction amongst users of psychoactive drugs. Otherwise there is a risk that an anti-drugs ideology may develop which might in its own way be as damaging as ideologies which insist on the medicalization of mental distress.

There are many progressive, radical and innovative perspectives on mental health within mainstream psychiatry and clinical psychology which stop short of directly challenging the positivist ideologies which have traditionally prevailed within those professions. For example, Carl Jung's ideas about psychosis in many ways prefigure the existentialist psychiatry of Laing and his colleagues. Similarly, the work of Laing and his colleagues at Kingsley Hall resonated with Maxwell Jones's work with groups in the British army and at the Henderson Unit, and David Clark's work in applying the therapeutic community approach to a large Victorian psychiatric hospital at Fulbourn. Disappointingly though, there is scant reference to these connections in the writings of Laing and his colleagues. Admittedly, this is a failing which is by no means exclusive to self-styled critics of psychiatry. A similar criticism could justifiably be made of the many cognitive therapists who are now suggesting symptoms of psychosis may be understood and managed without drugs. These ideas do not seem to be too far removed from the existentialist approach to psychoses advocated by Laing and his colleagues, but few cognitive therapists acknowledge that there is any connection (see Haddock and Slade, 1996).

The failure to acknowledge these connections is significant for two reasons. First, it represents failure to acknowledge the positive contributions made by mainstream medical psychiatrists and clinical psychologists to our understanding of mental distress and the compassionate treatment of distressed persons, both collectively and as individuals. The consequence of this oversight is that the critics have created a false dichotomy between those perspectives which are self-consciously radical and progressive and those which promote innovative practice within the context of mainstream mental health services. Thus, many followers of the critical theorists (although not necessarily the critical theorists themselves) have tended to demonize mainstream theory and practice and elevate their heroes to the level of all-knowing, all-powerful gurus. This is particularly evident in what Parker *et al.* (1995) have described as 'the Laing cult' – the existence of hard-core followers of Laing who find it difficult to accept any criticisms of their hero. For example, at least one reviewer of Adrian Laing's book about the life and work of his father seemed to have been offended by his cynicism about some aspects of his father's work and relationships with others. This is in spite of the fact that the book also includes warm affectionate memories which Adrian Laing has of his father (Hinchliffe, 1995: 38 cf. Laing, 1994). Similarly, other reviewers of books about Laing have overlooked the lack of methodological rigour in much of Laing's work, and have suggested that he was ignored solely because he challenged orthodoxy:

> He presented ... entirely empirical arguments and rebuttals. And of course, within the profession, he was entirely ignored ... Therapy as a sounding board. This made Laing a sort of secular priest ... A shaman, a sort of Western Zen master.
>
> (Virden, 1996: 46)

Second, the failure of critics of psychiatry to recognize the existence of critical and radical discourses within the mainstream (for example, therapeutic communities and other forms of social psychiatry) militates against their oppositional critiques being taken seriously by traditional psychiatrists and psychologists.

Throughout the history of British medical psychiatry it is possible to identify important humanitarian advances at both the structural and ideological levels. Medical psychiatry first began to emerge during the eighteenth century when humanitarian physicians such as William

Battie, Nathaniel Cotton and Thomas Withers became involved in the lucrative and often disreputable 'mad business'. They helped to transform the care of mentally distressed persons by emphasizing the importance of inter-personal relationships, occupational therapy and recruiting attendants who were patient and understanding (Nolan, 1993). Notwithstanding the introduction of a variety of unscientific and ineffective 'treatments' into mainstream psychiatry during the nineteenth century, the humanitarian ideals which underpinned the development of medical psychiatry continued to be evident. For example, medical supervision of inmates of asylums in England and Wales was originally introduced to protect them from physical and sexual abuse at the hands of attendants. It was the Medico-Psychological Association (later to become the Royal College of Psychiatrists) which in 1890 introduced a system of nurse training for asylum attendants as a way of raising standards of care (Nolan, 1993; Scull, 1993). More recently, medical psychiatry has contributed to the development of the phenothiazine drugs. Despite their well-known unpleasant side effects, the exaggerated claims made by their manufacturers and occasional misuse by clinicians, such drugs may have played a small but important part in enabling mental health professionals to develop new approaches to care. Ultimately they may have led to an improved quality of life for many people suffering severe mental distress (see Jones, 1993).

Critics of behavioural psychology have often overlooked the humanistic considerations that underpin the behavioural approach to therapy. The behaviour therapy that was widely practised in mental health and learning disability services during the 1970s was largely based on the work of B. F. Skinner (see Lanyon and Lanyon, 1978; Nursing Times Services, 1973; Wolpe, 1973). While conceding that behavioural psychology could be misinterpreted and misused Skinner argued that, because it considered only antecedents and consequences rather than states of mind, behavioural psychology was inherently non-judgemental and increased the freedom and dignity of human beings (Skinner, 1973). These claims have been contested (see Rogers, 1980). However, it is clear from Skinner's critique of punishment and his contention that all behaviour is learnt through reinforcement/reward (which implicitly challenges moralistic discourse of blame) that he was motivated by humanitarian considerations rather than by a sinister fascination with developing mechanisms of controlling human behaviour (see Skinner, 1973, 1974). Moreover, by the early 1990s the mechanistic approaches associated with behaviour modification programmes were no longer in vogue, having been displaced by more sophisticated cognitive-behavioural approaches. Significantly, cognitive-behavioural therapists have played an important role in promoting the treatment of some of the most severe forms of mental distress without recourse to medication (Bentall, 1992; Haddock and Slade, 1996; Kingdon and Turkington, 1995).

It is important not to demonize medical psychiatry or clinical psychology and to recognize that the vast majority of psychiatrists and clinical psychologists sincerely wish to alleviate the suffering experienced by mentally distressed persons. Certainly there are not many examples of psychiatrists contributing to the development of ground-breaking user-centred approaches to care and treatment, but neither are all mental health professionals megalomaniacs. Humanitarian considerations are frequently evident in the pages of many basic textbooks on medical psychiatry and clinical psychology. Although the cold, clinical descriptions of 'mental illnesses' and 'mental states' in these books often seem to lack empathy, sentiments such as those expressed in the following extract from a very traditional textbook of psychiatry are not uncommon in this literature:

> but there are [doctors] who say that they are too busy to listen to the complaints of their nervous patients, who dismiss them summarily ... but our view is that it is implicit in the doctor's calling and his obligation to relieve distress wherever he finds it irrespective of its psychological or physical nature; and it is his failure to do so which renders patients disappointed with orthodox medicine so that they turn, in despair, to the arts of the unqualified [*sic*].
> (Batchelor, 1969: 17)

At a structural level, medical psychiatry is implicated in a variety of policing and socio-political control mechanisms. Many of the ideological assumptions which prevail within both clinical psychology and medical psychiatry are not proven and contradict many distressed persons' understanding of their own experiences (see, for example, Harrison, 1995; Kitzinger and Perkins, 1993; Pembroke, 1994; Romme and Escher, 1993). In this sense, it is important that critiques of psychiatry and clinical psychology are taken seriously. On the other hand, critics of psychiatry and psychology who ignore any evidence which contradicts their own hypotheses and theories may impede the development of our understanding of mental distress by diverting our attention from other important discoveries and insights. That being said, positivist and medicalizing discourses of mental distress are flawed as they often tend to ignore evidence which shows that mental health and mental distress are affected by social and political circumstances. Furthermore, there is an inherent tendency in such approaches to objectify behaviour and experience and ignore emotional considerations.

Within mainstream psychiatry and psychology some of the most enlightening contributions to our understanding of mental distress are those which have been developed by individual psychoanalysts and psychiatrists who have experienced political oppression within their own lives. For example, the psychoanalysts Viktor Frankl and Bruno Bettelheim modified their own understanding of the human condition after being incarcerated in Nazi concentration camps (Bettelheim, 1986; Frankl, 1984). Similarly, Frantz Fanon's views about mental health were influenced by his experiences as a psychiatrist practising in Algeria during that country's war for independence from France (Fanon, 1967).

Less dramatically, psychiatrists whose work has been firmly located within mainstream medical psychiatry have pioneered some of the most innovative and progressive experiments in mental health care. Notable examples include the fusion of psychoanalysis and medical psychiatry practised at the Tavistock Clinic since the 1920s, and the therapeutic communities developed by Tom Main, Maxwell Jones, David Clark and others within National Health Service psychiatric hospitals between the 1950s and 1970s (see Clark, 1996; Kennard and Roberts, 1983; Mullan, 1995).

Significantly, the history of medical psychiatry is characterized by a selective eclecticism which has led to it incorporating psychoanalytical theories, cognitive-behavioural perspectives and therapeutic communities into the mainstream. In the field of clinical psychology, behaviour therapy (possibly influenced by the growth of interest in counselling and other talking therapies) has evolved into cognitive-behavioural psychotherapy. By contrast, there has been a tendency for critical theorists/practitioners to remain isolated from the mainstream and even from each other. Given their open hostility to medical psychiatry and clinical psychology, and some of the reactions of the establishment to them, their isolation from the mainstream is perhaps unsurprising. Their isolation from each other, however, is more difficult to explain. Certainly, there are tensions between [Thomas Szasz's right-wing critique of medical psychiatry and the existentialist psychiatrists' vaguely left-wing theories that mental distress is the product of particular forms of social organization, but there is common ground in both parties' rejection of medical psychiatry. However, although dialectical analysis of these overlaps and tensions might lead to a better understanding of the flaws in medical psychiatry, this has rarely been attempted. Instead, many writers conflate the views of Szasz and the existentialist anti-psychiatrists, while others acknowledge the differences between the two ideologies without exploring them.

It is unclear why this lack of intellectual rigour has been so commonplace amongst the critics of mainstream mental health services. Notwithstanding the lack of focus of some of his later work, Laing's first book *The Divided Self* was well written, intellectually rigorous and truly ground-breaking (Laing, 1959). Similarly, many of Thomas Szasz's books reflect high standards of scholarship. Nevertheless, even some of the most radical critics of mainstream ideologies of mental health have failed to debate alternative critical perspectives and/or to locate their work in the context of similar ideas which have been put forward by earlier writers.

One of the most striking examples of a critical theorist of mental health failing to acknowledge the links between his work and a previous writer is David Cooper's virtual disregard of the clinical psychiatry of Frantz Fanon. Cooper's ideas about mental health were explicitly socialist and existentialist, as were Fanon's. However, while Cooper publicly acknowledged his admiration of Fanon's anti-colonialist political philosophy, he made only passing reference to the connections between Fanon's politics and his (Fanon's) clinical practice (see Cooper, 1968). Similarly, in Elaine Showalter's feminist critique of psychiatry she criticizes Laing and Cooper for what she regards as their sexist attitudes to the distressed women who came into contact with them (Showalter, 1987). While Showalter's criticisms of Laing and Cooper in this respect may be justified, her distaste for this aspect of their behaviour prevents her from objectively evaluating the overlap between Cooper's theories about the role of nuclear families in contributing to mental distress, and the feminist critiques of nuclear families.

Further evidence of the lack of continuity between the various critical perspectives is to be found in the scant reference made to the work of Laing and Szasz by Jeffrey Masson in his uncompromising critique of all forms of psychotherapy. Indeed, in the case of Szasz, Masson adds insult to injury by boldly stating 'Perhaps the best known critic of psychiatry is Thomas Szasz. But he has not widened his criticism to psychotherapy' (1990: 229). In fact Szasz is the author of a book unambiguously entitled *The Myth of Psychotherapy* (Szasz, 1979a), which is in fact referenced elsewhere in Masson's book *Against Therapy* (1990). However, instead of offering a thorough critique of that book, Masson quotes selectively from a preface which Szasz wrote to another writer's book, in a way which seems to imply that Masson regards himself as being even more radical than Szasz. Maybe this is not what Masson intended, but it does suggest that he has missed an opportunity to develop his own critique in the context of work which had been developed earlier.

In this book we review various critical perspectives on mental health and mental distress; identify overlaps and tensions between the competing critical perspectives; and suggest a tentative model for the understanding of mental distress which takes account of such overlap and contradiction. However, as we have both been practitioners in mental health professions, we are all too aware of the dangers of producing neat theoretical models that are of little practical use. Thus, we recognize that many distressed persons and many mental health professionals continue to accept the legitimacy of many clinical practices which have been pilloried by critics of mainstream theories of mental health. Consequently, we accept that there may be circumstances in which psychotropic drugs can be used in a way which 'empowers' service users. For example, minor tranquillizers such as Valium (diazepam) and other benzodiazepines can be used very effectively to manage acute anxiety as *part of a wider strategy* of *short-term* crisis intervention (Hedaya, 1996). However, while we accept that medical psychiatry has made some important contributions to our understanding of mental distress, we have reservations about the use of electro-convulsive therapy (ECT) and psychosurgical interventions. This is because these interventions may not necessarily achieve the desired outcomes and carry a high risk of apparently irreversible side effects. On the other hand, one of us has seen severely depressed persons who have responded well to short courses of ECT and there are service users who willingly accept such treatment (see Perkins, 1999b). Nevertheless, there is a tendency for service users not to be given accurate information about how ECT works and what side effects there might be. Additionally, there are some clinicians who continue to regard it as a 'treatment of choice' for certain forms of mental distress despite the controversy surrounding its use. Psychosurgical interventions are even less easy to justify as they are, by definition, irreversible. Nevertheless, there may be exceptional circumstances where a person's mental distress is so incapacitating that psychosurgery might be a viable option. However, even then, it could only be justified if the *patient* genuinely believed that all other therapeutic options had been exhausted, and s/he had been given accurate and detailed information about all possible outcomes of any surgical procedures (including information about side effects, the likelihood of success/failure of any proposed procedure and other risks).

Notwithstanding these reservations, we acknowledge that it may be possible to develop socio-biological perspectives which are in some sense user-centred and empowering. For example, some biological psychiatrists argue that an understanding of mental distress which accepts that an individual might be biologically predisposed to behave in certain ways facilitates a more compassionate response to that person's situation (Hedaya, 1996). Thus the 'problem' is not necessarily with explanations which hold that some aspects of behaviour are biologically determined. Rather it lies with those medical practitioners who assume that this gives them the right to manipulate an individual's biochemistry in an attempt to control that person's behaviour, regardless of whether or not that person has consented to such intervention. Moreover, a truly critical perspective on mental health must be based on a consideration of all theoretical perspectives, and not just those which have been styled radical theories of mental health by those who have developed them.

The investigation of mental health and the development of intellectual ideas about mental health are complex tasks. While it is true that there is no incontrovertible evidence to either support or refute the proposition that mental health problems are 'illnesses' which may be diagnosed and treated like physical illnesses, there is unquestionably some relationship between body and mind. At its simplest, there are such phenomena as toxic confusional states and the well-known 'fight or flight' syndrome. The latter is the phenomenon whereby fear or anxiety results in certain autonomic nervous system reactions such as dilation of the pupils of the eyes, an increase in heart rate and release of adrenaline in order to prepare the body to deal with an external threat. More controversially there are holistic psychotherapeutic interventions which are based on the interaction of body and mind. These include Arthur Janov's primal therapy, Reichian therapeutics, psychosynthesis and the Alexander Technique (Capra, 1983; Farrell, 1991; Law, 1979). It would therefore seem to be naive to discount all of the theories associated with biological psychiatry.

This book is not intended to be a textbook which prescribes a 'correct' way to develop a critical approach to mental health care, and neither is it intended to offer a totally new paradigm for understanding mental health and mental distress. Rather, it is intended to suggest a way forward out of the ideological muddle that characterizes our understanding of mental health and mental distress at the beginning of the twenty-first century.

Despite over a hundred years of scientific research into the causation and treatment of mental distress, we are still unable to provide any incontrovertible evidence of either what causes mental distress or how it can be treated effectively. There is, though, a considerable body of circumstantial evidence which suggests that mental distress is the product of interplay between various psychological, social, political, environmental and biological factors. Regrettably, few mental health professionals are willing to take account of all these factors. Instead, many adopt one theoretical perspective and therapeutic approach as their own and disregard any new research findings which might challenge their beliefs. While such identity politics and celebration of difference are in keeping with the post-modernist *zeitgeist* of the late 1990s, it will not necessarily lead to us furthering our understanding of what causes mental distress, how to prevent it and how to respond to it. This book offers a critical review of our present understanding of mental health and mental distress and a tentative solution to the vexed question of how we might develop this understanding further.

We begin by evaluating the impact of advances in psychiatry and clinical psychology and psychotherapy and examining sociological critiques of the theory and practice of mental health care. From this starting point, mainstream ideas about mental health and mental distress and the strengths and shortcomings of statutory mental health services are evaluated.

Chapter 1 is a review of various historical perspectives on the emergence of British psychiatry in the nineteenth century. The aim is to identify and critically discuss the tensions and contradictions within and between such perspectives. In particular, the contribution of revisionist perspectives is acknowledged insofar as they provide an important counterbalance to traditional Whig accounts of the history of modern psychiatry. Additionally, recognition is given to the long history of contributions from users of mental health services in writing about their experiences as patients/clients of mental health professionals. Thus, the chapter sets the scene for what follows: a post-revisionist, post anti-psychiatry analysis of the theory and practice of mental health care which takes account of the sometimes competing perspectives of mental health professionals, users of mental health services and academics in the mental health field.

Chapter 2 offers a critical evaluation of some of the major changes affecting theory, policy and practice in mental health services throughout the twentieth century. In the earlier part of the century these included: the influence of the eugenics movement on the mental health professions, the shift from the asylums and custodial care to

psychiatric hospitals and therapeutic intervention, and experimentation with physical treatments such as insulin coma, ECT and
psychosurgery. Since the Second World War the most significant
development has been the gradual move towards community care. The
various factors contributing to the process of deinstitutionalization
are identified and analysed. The chapter concludes with an analysis of
the significance of medicalization in the development of mental health
theory, policy and practice throughout the twentieth century.

Chapter 3 is a critical analysis of some major theories of mental
distress which have been developed outside psychiatry; an exploration
of the extent to which they have been incorporated into psychiatric
practice; and consideration of the extent to which such therapeutic
approaches are consistent with user-centred mental health service
provision. The main perspectives discussed in this chapter are
psychoanalysis, behavioural psychology, Rogerian person-centred
psychotherapy and the self-help approaches favoured by some
sections of the mental health service users' movement. There are, of
course, many other approaches to the management of mental distress
but the significance of these particular perspectives is that they have
all had a profound effect on the way in which mainstream mental
health services in Britain have evolved. As there are so many other
schools of psychotherapy a comprehensive review of them all is
beyond the scope of this book. However, therapeutic approaches
which have enjoyed brief periods of being fashionable and/or well
known, such as Transactional Analysis and Gestalt Therapy, are also
discussed briefly. At the end of the chapter, the overlap and tension
between these various theories are discussed; and there is reference to
eclectic and skills-based models of counselling and psychotherapy.

Chapter 4 is an evaluation of the impact of the anti-psychiatry
movement and other direct critiques of mainstream ideologies of
mental health. The similarities and differences between the critiques
offered by Thomas Szasz and the so-called anti-psychiatrists are
explored, as is the impact of these ideas on mainstream mental health
services. In the final part of the chapter, the critical work which has
been developed in the late 1980s and early 1990s by Jeffrey Masson,
Peter Breggin and members of mental health service users' movements
is discussed in terms of the relationship of these ideas to the work of
the anti-psychiatry movement of the 1960s and 1970s (i.e. R. D.
Laing, David Cooper *et al.*), and the right-wing libertarian perspective
of Thomas Szasz.

Chapter 5 explores the significance of gender and race in the
development of ideas about mental health and mental distress. The

chapter begins with a review of the various contributions from within feminist theory and research regarding explanations for women's madness and women's experience of the mental health system. Key issues for the development of gender-sensitive mental health services are identified and evaluated. The chapter moves on to review the literature around race, ethnicity and mental distress, with particular reference to the distinction that has emerged between transcultural and anti-racist analyses. The significance of these debates is considered in relation to both the training of mental health professionals and innovations in mental health service delivery.

Chapter 6 consolidates the material developed in the first five chapters to argue that throughout its existence, psychiatry has been subjected to challenges to its legitimacy. These challenges have emerged from both within and outside its ranks and at a variety of levels – theoretical, technological, institutional and legislative. Key debates and issues at each of these levels are identified and discussed. The chapter culminates in an evaluation of the contemporary debates around risk, violence and dangerousness in mental health theory and practice and the perceived failure of care in the community for those in mental distress.

In Chapter 7 a theoretical approach borrowed from critical criminology is applied to the question of mental health/mental distress and the key characteristics of a critical perspective on mental health and mental distress are defined. The final chapter explores the implications for practice of the analysis developed in Chapter 7.

1   The historical maze

Nowadays the significance of historical analysis to critical theory and research is rarely disputed. However obvious this assumption, it has to be recognized that there are serious difficulties involved in interpreting and evaluating contemporary theories and practices in mental health with reference to the past. Not least among these difficulties is the existence of multiple 'histories' – of psychiatry and its allied disciplines; of 'madness' and its meanings; and of institutional responses to the 'mad' (Andrews *et al.*, 1997; Berrios and Freeman, 1991; Busfield, 1986; Bynum *et al.*, 1985a, 1985b, 1988; Gittins, 1998a; Hunter and MacAlpine, 1963; Jones, 1972, 1993; MacDonald, 1981; Nolan, 1993; Parry-Jones, 1972; Porter, 1987a, 1987b; Russell, 1997; Scull, 1979, 1981, 1989, 1993; Showalter, 1987; Skultans, 1975). In this respect any notion of a unified history of mental health theory and practice is something of a chimera.

The basis of the confusion is both methodological and conceptual. It relates not only to *how* people go about recording and researching data, but also to the particular *ideas and perspectives* they bring to the task. As Scull (1989: 3) notes, 'most historians, after all, quite rightly see themselves as engaged in the task of *explaining* and not just reproducing the past'. When searching for relevant contextual material it is usually necessary to rely on the painstaking work of others. In doing so, it has to be acknowledged that significantly different versions of historical 'reality' will be encountered. Nor is this problem easily overcome by conducting one's own archival research. Such a task is equally daunting and throws up its own dilemmas. 'History' is not some kind of storehouse of pure, uncontaminated 'truths' simply waiting for the contemporary researcher to uncover their significance for the present. Historical events, documents or artefacts cannot be understood devoid of messy context – be it social, cultural, economic, political, ideological or religious. Moreover, historical analysis is an inherently hazardous undertaking for contemporary generations of researchers engaging in acts of interpretation, as the attribution of meaning and intention to an historical event or account is a profoundly subjective exercise (Miller, 1994). That is, there are not merely difficulties to do with the recording of 'facts', but also to do with the conflicting views of society held by different historical researchers (Crotty, 1998; May and Williams, 1998; Outhwaite, 1987).

In the process of researching historical material for this text we have been struck by the enormous diversity of ways in which the history of ideas, institutions and practices has been represented by and for each generation. Layer upon layer of subjective meanings and interpretations have been constructed around this topic, making it almost impossible to trace a path through what we have come to call 'the historical maze' of psychiatry. Such is the sense of disorientation and fragmentation at times that it is difficult to know where to begin. Nevertheless, what follows is a survey of existing written histories of psychiatry, identifying points of tension and contradiction in the various perspectives. The intention is to draw out the significance of all contributions to an understanding of the dynamics of change in the theory and practice of mental health care.

The end of consensus

It is usually agreed that the 1960s, and the emergence of what have been termed the 'revisionist' historians, represent a critical turning point in psychiatric historiography. Their entry into the arena has to be understood in the wider context of the development of two crucial phenomena – the crisis in science and the crisis in society (Reinharz, 1993). By the late 1960s, the growth of symbolic interactionism, phenomenology and neo-Marxism had shaken the British positivistic empirical tradition to its roots (Craib, 1992; Waters, 1994). These perspectives emphasized the value of the individual experiences, subjectivity and personal autonomy of those being researched. They were also committed to exposing the significance of power relationships in the research process. The quest for the discovery of 'knowledge' or 'truth' in social scientific research had been dominated by the privileging of objectivity over subjectivity, of 'hard' over 'soft' data. Increasingly the appropriateness of the scientific method for understanding the complexities of social reality was questioned by critics who insisted on addressing the political, ethical, subjective and reflexive nature of social inquiry (Kuhn, 1962). This epistemological crisis went hand in hand with the massive social upheavals of the 1960s and 1970s. New social movements began to articulate the subjectivity/objectivity relation as political. Institutional power structures were shown to be closely associated with the ideologies and content of knowledge.

In the mental health field the 1967 *Congress on the Dialectics of Liberation*, organized by the members of the Philadelphia Association, was of great significance. The Congress was a forum in which existential psychiatrists, anarchists, Marxist intellectuals and political leaders met to discuss key social issues, representing a unique expression of the politics of dissent (Mullan, 1995). Prior to this, however, a variety of forces from within and outside clinical practice had emerged to challenge traditional psychiatric theory and practice (Goffman, 1961; Laing, 1959; Szasz, 1961). While they converged around negating the established doctrines of medical psychiatry, representing 'a tendency of opposition' (Sedgwick, 1982: 22), they diverged considerably in theoretical emphasis and in prescriptions for changes in practice (see Chapter 4 for a fuller discussion of some of these perspectives). Collectively, however, they exposed the inadequacy of the positivistic framework for understanding mental distress. All concurred that 'mental illness' is to a large extent socially caused or socially constructed. /They questioned whether the purpose of psychiatric 'treatment' is more to do with maintaining social order than the relief of suffering; and asserted that the dominance of the medical profession is neither warranted nor desirable (Ingleby, 1983).

This climate cultivated a rich cross-fertilization of ideas and methods between the disciplines of history and sociology, so that alongside the broader critiques of mainstream psychiatric knowledge and practice, a wave of historical writing emerged which represented a fundamental challenge to conventional accounts of the history of psychiatry (Castel, 1976; Doerner, 1981; Foucault, 1967; Rothman, 1971; Scull, 1979). These writers forced a re-examination of changing ideas and practices towards the insane, particularly during the eighteenth and nineteenth centuries – the so-called 'Golden Age' of psychiatry (Castel, 1976). Although, as with other critics of psychiatry and mental health services, they do not constitute a unified position, nevertheless their work as a whole shares some important ideas. First, that the process of identifying and responding to 'madness' is a culture-bound activity. Second, that what constitutes 'madness' is changeable and uncertain. Third, that 'mad' people, psychiatrists and psychiatric institutions must be understood in their sociological context. Finally, that psychiatrists have constructed versions of the past which are narrow and constricted, and thereby distorted (Scull, 1989). Such ideas have opened up provocative questions and heated debates in the study of mental health.

The 'Golden Age' of reform

In dealing with the history of mental health the most obvious organizing principle is chronological. Roy Porter (1987a) suggests that although contemporary histories of psychiatry differ in their interpretations, they nevertheless adhere to a common timeline. This usually begins in the late eighteenth century with the development of psychiatry (as a body of theory, a profession and a system of institutions) within an overarching legislative framework. There is a general consensus that during the first half of the eighteenth century the majority of the insane were to be found in the community, either at home or boarded out under the Poor Law, as there was as yet no formal segregation of the mad in England. The minority who were confined could be found in gaols, bridewells or one of the flourishing private, profit-oriented madhouses. These were run by people from various backgrounds, some mere speculators, others representative of more 'respectable' groups such as the clergy or the medical profession. The level of understanding of mental distress at this time was 'marked by a traditional mingling of magical, religious and scientific concepts. Individual cases of mental disorder might be attributed to divine retribution, diabolical possession, witchcraft, astrological influences, humoral imbalances, or to any combination of these forces' (MacDonald, 1981: 7). According to Jones (1993), superstition, moral condemnation, ignorance and apathy were the attitudes that dominated the treatment of mental disorder in the eighteenth century and, unsurprisingly, these were reflected in the pattern of administration.

By the middle of the nineteenth century, however, the picture was very different. The mad were clearly identified as a distinctive 'problem population' and were segregated in formal state institutions called asylums. Their condition was essentially seen as a medical problem and their care and treatment was overseen by a new group of professionals – 'mad doctors'. In 1800 there had been but a few thousand mad people confined in a variety of *ad hoc* establishments. By 1900 there were some 100,000 people confined in state asylums. In just one hundred years a major historical shift had occurred in society's response to the mad. The events surrounding this development are variously interpreted as representative of either:

- a 'march of progress' from the gloomy days of indifference, neglect and brutality towards a more enlightened 'moral' approach characterized by the application of science, humanitarianism and benevolence;
- an exercise in social control motivated by the emergence of the modern state in capitalist societies and/or medical imperialism;
- a complex dynamic involving elements of both of these positions (though more accidental than conspiratorial) producing unintentionally repressive consequences.

The 'history of good intentions' traces a steady path of reform from the days when the mad were either left to roam, uncared-for or subjected to exploitation and maltreatment in the disparate range of institutions that predated the 'curative' asylums of the late eighteenth and early nineteenth centuries. It is suggested that the sheer force of human misery pricked a new social conscience and sparked off a philanthropic impulse. Individuals concerned with the abuses and potential abuses of the private madhouse system began experimenting with more humane methods of care and treatment. Charitable institutions soon sprang up in many cities such as London, Manchester, York, Newcastle, Liverpool, Leicester and Exeter. The efforts and innovations of individual progressive reformers such as William Battie at St Luke's Asylum in London; the Tukes (William and Samuel) and the Jepsons (George and Katherine) at the York Retreat; Robert Gardiner Hill at the Lincoln County Asylum; W. A. F. Browne at Crichton Royal Asylum; and John Conolly at the Hanwell Asylum, are represented as benign manifestations of humanitarian concern. They are seen as indicative of the emergence of a more sophisticated view of the mad, not as brutes or animals, but in essence human beings suffering from a condition that was not their fault. With the promise of restorative cures through a system of 'moral treatment' and a commitment to 'non-restraint', these pioneers propelled central and local government towards a cascade of legislative reforms culminating in the 1845 Lunacy Act and the setting up of a mandatory system of public asylums.

'Moral treatment' was both something more and something less than 'the triumph of humanism and of therapy, a recognition that kindness, reason and tactful manipulation were more effective in dealing with the inmates of asylums than were fear, brutal coercion and restraint, and medical therapy' (Bynum in Scull, 1989: 83). It was no longer believed that the insane were *totally* deprived of their reason. Indeed moral treatment was aimed at appealing to their residual reason. The asylum was portrayed as a technical, objective response to the patient's condition, an environment that would provide the best possible conditions for recovery. It was to provide the insane with a sanctuary from a world in which they could not cope. However, the small intimate institution devoted to the cure and humane care of its residents did not translate so easily into the public domain. The new state asylums did not live up to expectations and conditions grew steadily worse as the numbers of inmates swelled. Whether because of residual problems associated with the 'old' regimes, or a failure to implement the new regime effectively, the new 'humane' approaches of moral therapy and non-restraint soon proved to be no more effective in curing insanity than the standard 'remedies' of bleeding, purging, blistering and vomiting. Nevertheless, the assumption prevailed that the dynamic of scientific progress was underway and that in the expert hands of medical men things could only continue to improve.

Clearly such accounts of the emergence of modern psychiatry represent mental distress as a technical–medical problem which will eventually be solved with the steady application of science (Ingleby, 1981; Pilgrim, 1992a). They dominated social histories of psychiatry up until the revisionist challenges of the 1960s and 1970s, and indeed have been defended and reasserted by some notable contemporary traditionalists (see Clare, 1976; Jones, 1972, 1993; Wing, 1978). By contrast, the revisionists are highly sceptical about the aims, beliefs and intentions of the reformers, arguing that they should not be taken at face value. They have sought to locate 'reform' in the social, economic and political contexts of the period, problematizing the relationship between intentions and consequences.

The 'Golden Age' revisited

Michel Foucault's (1961) pioneering work *Histoire de la folie a l'age classique* (*Madness and Civilisation*, 1967) laid the foundations for a critical review of psychiatric history. Often referred to as a 'prehistory' of psychiatry, Foucault's thesis affords a central position to what he calls 'the Great Confinement' throughout Europe during the Classical Age (1660–*c*1800), whereby the mad were rounded up and confined in an 'undifferentiated mass' (in Porter, 1987a: 6) along with paupers, criminals and beggars. He argues that this process was expedited through the breakdown of the dialogue between reason and unreason. That is until this point madness had enjoyed a liberty and truth of its own, but rationality dictated that it be disqualified and negated as 'unreason'. For Foucault it was during this period that the conditions were established under which the profession of psychiatry would eventually emerge in the late eighteenth and early nineteenth centuries. In this sense he sets the stage for the emergence of the psychiatric profession and leaves it to others to take up the story. He emphasizes the significance of Pinel in France and Tuke in England and the rise of 'moral treatment' as marking the moment when 'the medical gaze secures its domination of the mad' (Scull, 1989: 16). This is a far cry from the traditionally held romantic view of the reformers liberating the mad from iron shackles and physical barbarism. Foucault argues that their efforts constituted no improvement since moral treatment merely represented moral imprisonment and thereby 'madness mastered'. There was no longer the necessity for physical constraint since conformity could be achieved through a discourse of benevolent interventions:

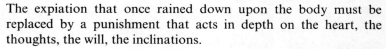

> The expiation that once rained down upon the body must be replaced by a punishment that acts in depth on the heart, the thoughts, the will, the inclinations.
>
> (Foucault, 1977: 16)

While Foucault's thesis represents an important counterbalance to the self-congratulatory, 'public relations' versions of psychiatric history, it is not unproblematic and indeed has since been repudiated, not least by Foucault himself (Miller, 1994). In particular there are issues of factual inaccuracy. For example, it has been acknowledged that Foucault's account is at variance with the facts for England, particularly regarding the scale of confinement of the mad during this period. Although the process of institutionalization had begun it was minuscule when compared with the developments of the second half of the nineteenth century (Porter, 1987a). Furthermore, Foucault's argument that 'the Great Confinement' was an exercise in the state suppression of anarchy does not stand up to scrutiny. In England there was no uniform centralized effort to manage the mad during the seventeenth or eighteenth centuries rather what provision existed was *ad hoc* and unsystematic. Furthermore, the relatively few who were confined were not only paupers but also significant numbers of the middle and upper classes. Porter (1987a) suggests that it was precisely this rich clientele who made the private 'trade in lunacy' so attractive and lucrative. Foucault has also been accused of romanticizing conditions during the Middle Ages. Clearly any notion of the mad roaming free and unhindered about the countryside must be tempered by the harsh truth that they were often beaten up, locked up or left to rot during this period (Scull, 1989).

Ingleby (1983) argues that *Madness and Civilisation* was really the starting point for Foucault's wider project of asserting the inextricable link between power and knowledge (see Foucault, 1972, 1980). It has been this aspect of his work which has proven to be of more lasting value and impact on critical research and writing in the mental health field (see, for example, Parker *et al.*, 1995). Nevertheless, *Madness and Civilisation* inspired a new generation of critical historians of mental health who, in the main, have been keen to avoid the Foucauldian tendency towards excessive romanticism and cavalier over-generalization. These authors highlighted the need for a more careful analysis of the reality of change (Porter, 1987a, 1987b; Scull, 1979, 1981, 1989, 1993).

For Andrew Scull (1993: 3) the process of 'reform' in psychiatry is 'embedded in far more complex ways in broader transformations of the English political and social structure'. He places more emphasis on the economic necessity of segregation than Foucault, identifying changes in the relations of production as underpinning changes in the pattern of provision for the insane. He does not infer a reductive, overly deterministic process of change, but rather a complex set of inter-relationships between social, economic and political forces; the professional aspirations of mad doctors; and 'a change in the cultural meaning of madness' (Scull, 1981: 108). Scull suggests that there should not be an uncritical acceptance of the reformers' accounts of their activities. Like Foucault he offers an examination of 'moral treatment's less benevolent aspects and its latent potential (all too soon realized) for deterioration into a repressive form of moral management' (Scull, 1981: 81). He sees the consequence of their efforts (whatever their intentions) as facilitating huge increase in the numbers of those incarcerated in a vast network of 'museums of madness' rather than improving the lot of those already incarcerated. In this sense he sees the reformers as providing an all too convenient solution to the problem of insanity for the new economic order.

Whereas the rise of the psychiatric profession is seen by the traditionalists as a consolidation of the reformers' gains, revisionists like Scull have exposed the realities of contradiction and conflict in the relationship between the medical men and the reformers regarding the care and treatment of the insane. Scull argues that the medical profession was barely interested in insanity until, during the middle of the eighteenth century, a number of doctors realized the profits to be made in the private mad-trade. This suggests that their motivations and intentions went beyond a straightforward desire to improve the treatment of the insane. For Scull, the entry of highly respected medical men into what was essentially considered to be the dubious and disreputable mad-business, marked a significant effort to claim insanity as a part of the legitimate domain of medicine. He concludes, 'doctors were gradually acquiring a dominant, although not a monopolistic position in the mad-business by the end of the eighteenth century' (1993: 185).

However, Scull notes that the emergence of the reform movement and moral treatment threatened to undermine medicine's claims to jurisdiction over the insane:

> Those laymen who ... had been agitating for lunacy reform on humanitarian grounds but who had previously lacked a viable alternative model ... eagerly seized on moral treatment.
>
> (1989: 132)

Scull argues that moral treatment posed a potential obstacle to the aspirations of the medical men through its apparent rejection of standard medical techniques. He describes the ensuing conflict in Parliament between the mad-doctors and the reformers during the first half of the nineteenth century. The latter sought to curb the authority of the medics by insisting on a strict system of lay administration and emphasizing the humanitarian value of 'non medical', moral therapy. In response the medical men made a case that only *they* could and should have the power to supervise patients' treatment. Indeed the 1828 Madhouse Act gave official recognition of the role of the medical profession in the management of the mad solely on the basis that they were the most appropriately qualified persons to safeguard the *physical* well-being of patients. They not only emphasized their long tradition and experience of administering the asylums, but also increasingly established all the trappings of expertise which would ensure their virtual monopoly status over the care and treatment of the insane. The Association of Medical Officers of Asylums and Hospitals for the Insane was founded in 1841 and its journal *The Asylum Journal* was founded in 1853.

These developments were clearly grounded in the wider context of a burgeoning scientism. Nolan notes:

> Growing up alongside an expanding and flourishing industrial society was the belief that health could be made available to all through the interventions of science ... Not only were physical

illnesses to be tackled and vanquished by science, but also those less tangible and more disturbing ailments of the mind.

(1993: 8)

After failing to oust the new regime the medical men opted to turn it to their advantage. Scull observes that since Tuke and his followers had no pretensions to professional status and had adhered to much of the existing medical language, moral treatment was vulnerable to takeover bids by the medical profession. He notes that 'in the absence of any rival helping group, medicine set about assimilating moral treatment within its own sphere of competence' (1993: 200). Scull's position synthesizes economic arguments to explain the rise of the asylum system with an examination of professional power struggles to account for the emergence of medical psychiatry's dominance of that system:

> A dialectical process was at work whereby the separation of the insane into madhouses and asylums helped to create the conditions for the emergence of an occupational group laying claim to expertise in their care and cure, and the nature and content of the restorative ideal which the latter fostered reinforced the commitment to the institutional approach.
>
> (1979: 44)

Clearly, Scull's thesis is in the company of a whole range of broader theoretical critiques analysing the social control functions of psychiatry and the medicalization of madness (Baruch and Treacher, 1978; Cohen, 1990; Ingleby, 1981; Miller and Rose, 1986; Rose, 1990; Szasz, 1961, 1963, 1971, 1990, 1994). These are discussed more fully in Chapter 2. Such approaches have been criticized for their implicit (or in some cases explicit) assumption that the actions and motivations of the reformers were disingenuous, rather than the genuine expression of humanitarian ideals (Nolan, 1993). Other studies have emerged within the revisionist tradition that have been less specifically concerned with theorizing the social control of the mad. Rather they have provided detailed searching re-examinations of the history of particular institutions and significant individuals (see, for example, Andrews et al., 1997; Digby, 1985; Tomes, 1988; Turner, 1988) rather than the critical wide-ranging surveys of history characterized by Foucault or Scull.

Roy Porter (1987a) warns against what he considers to be overly conspiratorial theories of social control of the mad. Of greater significance, he suggests, is the observation that prior to the nineteenth century the resources and institutions had not yet been developed which would have permitted a single professional group to assume full legal control of the mad. He is keen to challenge those versions of the history of psychiatry which identify a watershed at the beginning of the nineteenth century. Foucault (1967), Scull (1979) and some Whig historians have suggested that this period marked a change in the cultural meaning of madness; an impulse towards reform and a new therapeutic approach – i.e. moral treatment. Rather, Porter emphasizes continuities with the past, particularly with eighteenth century ideas and initiatives. He argues that much of what the nineteenth century claimed for its own had already been established by 'embryonic professional psychiatrists' (1987a: 173) such as William Battie. Battie's (1758) *Treatise on Madness*, Porter argues, contains the key ideas of moral therapy and stimulated new approaches to treating the mad in advance of Tuke and his followers. Porter offers a welcome counterbalance to Scull's scepticism regarding the intentions and contributions of reformers such as Battie. He also challenges those who have demonized eighteenth century ideas and practices in mental health care, arguing that at this time attitudes to the mad were characterized by diversity and individualism. This means that while there are horror stories of the insane being left naked, manacled, in filth and dehumanized, these experiences were not universal. Indeed, he cites evidence of the existence of establishments that were clean, in good order and at the forefront of humanitarian interventions.

Of particular significance in Porter's work is a concern to recognize the contributions of the mad themselves to psychiatric historiography. The voices of the mad, he suggests, have been conspicuously absent from most accounts. This has a resonance with the argument in Foucault (1967) that during the eighteenth century the mad were 'silenced'. Porter (1987a: 236) comments, 'in any case, psychiatric theory advised that delusion was contagious and that it was foolish to reason with the mad'. It is not surprising then to find that there is very little documentary evidence of people's experiences of these early interventions – particularly before the nineteenth century. Nevertheless, Porter brings to our attention some of the few available narratives and emphasizes their value as communications in their own right:

The writings of the mad challenge the discourse of the normal, challenge its right to be the objective mouthpiece of the times. The assumption that there exists definitive and unitary standards of truth and falsehood, reality and delusion, is put to the test.

(1987b: 3)

Such an approach reflects the valorization of individual experience, identity, and subjectivity so characteristic of the phenomenological approaches of the 1960s, and the psychiatric user movements of the 1970s and 1980s (see Chapter 4 for a fuller discussion of these perspectives).

Although few in number and prone to the same limitations outlined at the beginning of this chapter (particularly since all are written by highly articulate men), the autobiographical accounts cited in Porter (1987a, 1987b) provide an important dimension to any understanding of the process of change during the eighteenth and nineteenth centuries. As well as producing written accounts of their experiences and views, they frequently petitioned Parliament, calling for investigations and changes in legislation and practices (for example those such as Louisa Lowe, Urbane Metcalf, John Mitford, Richard Paternoster and John Perceval). Additionally, there were a number of campaigning organizations comprised of patients and their allies, such as the Alleged Lunatics' Friend Society, the Friends of Insane Persons and the Society for the Protection of Alleged Lunatics. Thus, it is important to observe that 'the history of patient protest ... roughly parallels the history of asylum reform' (Peterson, 1977: 151).

The earliest accounts, drawn from the second half of the seventeenth century, appear to support the argument that people were for the most part left free to be mad and that very little in the way of 'psychiatric' intervention occurred at all. By the eighteenth century the accounts are dominated by 'the madhouse' and indicate that the writers saw themselves as prisoners not patients. That is their main complaints focused on their experiences of social exclusion and removal from their families and communities rather than on any psychiatric regime as such. Certainly such dissent was felt on a much wider scale and fuelled public pressure for action to prevent wrongful confinement. This culminated in the introduction of 1774 Act for Regulating Private Madhouses. Attention at this time appears to be directed towards individual cases of injustice rather than general issues concerning the quality of care and treatment of the insane. By the nineteenth century the focus is not on unlawful confinement or cruelty but 'treatment' itself. John Perceval's attack on the Ticehurst and Brislington asylums (then considered two of the most respected establishments) gives a very different interpretation of 'moral therapy' than that of progressive, humane psychiatry. He refers to it as a 'brutal and tyrannical control over my will' (cited in Porter, 1987a: 272). Porter (1987a: 273) says that from this point onwards 'the history of mad people's writing is a crescendo of reaction to, and protest against, the dominating presence of the asylum'. In this sense, he suggests, their writing bears out the truth of the 'rising presence of the asylum and of psychological medicine as the framework which increasingly defined and mastered madness'.

In a similar vein to Porter, Elaine Showalter's (1987) *The Female Malady: Women, Madness and English Culture, 1830–1980*, is characteristic of scholarship which has sought to give prominence to the subjective experiences of those on the receiving end of psychiatry rather than the history of institutions, ideas and the profession itself. Drawing on a rich array of sources – paintings, photographs, film, asylum records, oral histories – Showalter contributes an innovative gendered dimension to the study of psychiatric historiography. For Showalter, psychiatry's treatment of women is firmly located in the context of a patriarchal social order. (A fuller discussion of Showalter and other feminist critiques of psychiatry are developed in Chapter 3.) She explores popular and professional discourses about the relationship between women and madness, arguing that madness became a distinctively female condition during the first half of the nineteenth century. Mad-doctors constructed elaborate explanations to argue for women's greater susceptibility to insanity. In particular it was women's reproductive organs that were identified as the source of their mental distress and the focus of drastic 'treatments' such as clitoridectomy:

> English psychiatric treatment of nervous women was ruthless, a microcosm of the sex war intended to establish the male doctor's total authority.
>
> (Showalter, 1987: 137)

Showalter discusses how the burgeoning diagnosis of hysteria came to epitomize all manifestations of female madness. Moreover, she notes that as the asylum population expanded, sex ratios started to change with more women (particularly poor women) being confined than men, so that, 'by the end of the century, women had decisively taken the lead as psychiatric patients, a lead they have retained ever since, and in ever-increasing numbers' (1987: 52). Although she has been criticized for exaggerating the statistical significance of this gendered imbalance and at times romanticizing women's mental distress, Andrew Scull considers Showalter's work apt and insightful. He notes:

> The assertion that our culture somehow equates madness and the female species is not without foundation; and our organized responses to these maladies repeatedly turn out to be influenced, in ways both gross and subtle, by questions of sexuality and gender.
>
> (1989: 271)

From the various perspectives outlined above it is evident that a simplistic approach to the history of psychiatry is heavily problematic. As David Rothman (in Cohen and Scull, 1983: 117) argues, 'it is too complicated to allow for "either-or" approaches. It is not a question of reform *or* social control, ideology *or* reality'. What is clear, however, is that while the reformers pioneered changing conceptions of insanity and its treatment, their ideas did not spring up in a vacuum. Without the revisionist contributions this fact would almost certainly have remained obscured:

> Whatever the excesses and inadequacies of the various revisionist accounts of lunacy reform, one must surely be grateful to them for liberating us from the narrowness and naivete of a vision that reduced the whole process to a simplistic equation: humanitarianism + science + government inspection = the success of 'the great nineteenth century movement for a more humane and intelligent treatment of the insane'.
>
> (Scull, 1989: 34)

While the second half of the nineteenth century was a decisive period in the history of psychiatry, the position of the asylum doctors continued to be somewhat paradoxical. Although they had consolidated their claims *vis-à-vis* responsibility for treating insanity, their activities were still constrained by a complex legal and administrative framework. For example, a number of non-medical reformers fuelled anxieties about the possibility of illegal confinement, insisting on closer legal scrutiny and authority over the process of certification. Such concerns led to the 1890 Lunacy Act which enhanced judicial powers over certification of the insane. The Act gave priority to legal controls and safeguards over medical opinion thereby hindering the medical men's ambitions in relation to early treatment. Additionally, the relative isolation of the asylum doctors from the general medical profession meant that there were significant physical boundaries to their power and influence. While the asylums became more custodial than curative in character, filling up with chronic cases of society's unwanted, a new breed of asylum doctors was emerging with their own claims to special expertise. Imitating broader developments in the medical sphere, the emphasis was on the brain, the importance of heredity and the value of systems of classification. Nevertheless, it was primarily outside of the asylum that new disease categories, new forms of treatment and new professional alliances were being developed which would propel psychiatry into the twentieth century.

2 From asylum to community
Relocating psychiatry

A number of inter-related themes have underpinned the development of psychiatry during the twentieth century. First, its influence and activities have spread beyond the asylum. The structure of mental health services has been transformed from the large-scale nineteenth century custodial asylums, set apart from the community, to incorporate a diverse range of publicly funded services within the community (Busfield, 1986, 1996). However, the extent to which the transition from institutional to community psychiatry has been adequately supported by appropriate organizational and financial resources continues to be a matter of debate. Second, the focus of psychiatric theory and practice has become increasingly diverse, both in terms of the type of problem receiving attention and the character of those being treated. There has been a broadening of categories of mental disorder, in particular the psychoneuroses, and a concentration on acute rather than chronic problems. This has been accompanied by a growth in voluntary 'therapeutic' relationships rather than coercive treatment; an increasing emphasis on mental health as a public health issue; and a mushrooming industry in 'alternative' models of intervention such as counselling and psychotherapy (Pilgrim and Rogers, 1993). Third, and closely related to the last point, is the diversity of other mental health professions which have emerged throughout the century. Although in law it is the psychiatrist who has primary clinical responsibility for the care and treatment of the mentally disordered, to a great extent this professional dominance has been constrained by the development of the psychiatric *team* with its eclectic range of skills in psychiatry, psychology, social work, nursing and occupational therapy.

Each of these themes will be evident in the following examination of the broader transformations in mental health theory, policy and practice during the twentieth century. However, it is not so easy to trace a discrete path of evolutionary ideas in mental health theory, policy and practice without again encountering messy contradictions. As Prior (1993: 48) warns, 'the history of twentieth century psychiatry does not lend itself to the drawing of simple divisions, nor to the display of any easily readable trends away from one set of objects and locations and towards another'.

The Victorian legacy

During the first decades of the twentieth century the character of the public asylum changed very little. Scull's bleak vision of 'museums of madness' gives apt expression to the sense of decline in the whole profession at the time. It is an era that was reflected on by Ernest Jones as 'Chubb lock psychiatry' indicating 'the low level at which their (psychiatrists) branch of medicine subsisted' (in Turner, 1988: 152). The asylum system had drawn all manner of social outcasts into it. Heavily influenced by the eugenic ideas of Francis Galton, early biological psychiatry elaborated degeneracy theory, linking together the mad, the bad and the inadequate. In *Hereditary Genius* (1869) and *Natural Inheritance* (1889) Galton argued that just like physical attributes such as eye or hair colour, mental abilities and character were inherited. The implication of this, and what caused most concern, was the notion that *social* degeneracy – insanity, criminality, illegitimacy, alcoholism and pauperism – could be transmitted from generation to generation. It was argued that a whole range of socially undesirable behaviours could be explained by a tainted gene pool in the lower social classes. Most forms of mental deficiency and mental illness were assumed to have hereditary origins with little distinction between the two categories of disorder being made at this time. Thus both insanity and 'feeble-mindedness' were considered to be key elements in this degeneration as illustrated in Henry Goddard's work on *The Kallikak Family*:

> We have here a family of good English blood ... throughout four generations maintaining a reputation for honour and respectability of which they are justly proud. Then a scion of this family, in an unguarded moment, steps aside from the paths of rectitude and, with the help of a feeble-minded girl, starts a line of mental defectives that is truly appalling. After this mistake, he returns to the traditions of his family, marries a woman of his own quality, and through her carries on a line of respectability equal to that of his ancestors.
>
> (in Sapsford, 1981: 315)

However, as Prior (1993: 128) notes, 'madness was believed to result from hereditary causes long before any systematic scientific theory of hereditary transmission was available, and well before any empirical evidence for such a belief was collected'. Indeed the primary evidence used by Galton, Goddard and their contemporaries to support their assertions was *statistical* not biological. Nevertheless, these mistaken beliefs encouraged some interested parties (most notably the eugenicists) to argue for the isolation of the mentally deficient and mentally ill. Since they were considered to be sexually permissive and prolific in producing defective offspring, 'curbing their reproduction, by segregation or sterilization was a matter of urgency, and hence their detection and ascertainment was a priority' (Rose, 1989: 136).

Social policies soon began to reflect these concerns. For example, the *Royal Commission on the Care of the Feeble-minded (1904–8)* heard evidence from various individuals and groups preoccupied with the fear of a declining national stock. These included some of the most influential philanthropic and charitable organizations of the time such as the Charity Organisation Society and The Salvation Army. Since the term 'feeble-minded' was so ill defined the discussions of the Commission ranged over the many aspects of social degeneracy. It considered compulsory sterilization, but drew back from recommending this as official policy. Instead, it attempted to follow a middle line between preserving the liberty of the subject and taking heed of eugenic theory by advocating permanent segregation. Under the *Mental Deficiency Act* of 1913 the 'mentally defective' were categorized into four 'types' – 'idiots', 'imbeciles', 'feeble-minded persons' and 'moral imbeciles'. This piece of legislation reflected accelerated efforts by the early psychiatrists to emulate their peers in physical medicine by classifying and categorizing human behaviour into rigid 'scientific' systems. Yet the social problems of criminality, illegitimacy, pauperism, insanity and feeble-mindedness were frequently inter-mingled and explanations for them were put forward in both medical and moral terms. Moreover, the processes surrounding definition, diagnosis and classification were permeated with prevailing ideologies based on pejorative assumptions about race, class and gender (see Chapter 5 for a full discussion of these critiques). For example, under the Act any unmarried woman in receipt of poor relief who gave birth to a child would be labelled a 'moral imbecile'. The control of the 'dangerous sexuality' of working-class women represented an essentially racist state policy aimed at preventing the deterioration of 'the great British stock' (O'Malley and Hall, 1990).

In its most extreme form eugenics underpinned policies of mass extermination and sterilization of 'racially inferior' groups in Nazi Germany, along with the physically and mentally disabled (Burleigh, 1994). Yet the basic suppositions of German eugenic medicine were essentially the same as those touted in Britain and the USA. Assumptions about genetic and racial inferiority are thus deeply embedded in Western psychiatric theory. By the end of the nineteenth century the myth that the brains of black people were smaller than those of whites was commonly accepted (Fernando, 1988; Thomas and Sillen, 1972). The so-called 'founding fathers' of psychiatry and psychology all peddled degeneracy theory and added their own particular variation on the theme. For example, the psychologist Stanley Hall described Asians, Chinese, Africans and indigenous Americans as psychologically 'adolescent races'; the prominent British psychiatrist Henry Maudsley and the psychoanalyst Sigmund Freud both argued that black people were relatively immune to mental illness because they lacked civilization, while others said they were mentally degenerate because they lacked Western culture. By the 1930s Carl Jung was theorizing 'racial infection', warning people of the psychological dangers of living too close to blacks (Fernando, 1988).

So often these ideas were intertwined with crude pre-occupations about the sexuality of non-white races and the insane. Henry Maudsley, who was obsessed with masturbation, wrote of 'the miserable sinner whose mind suffers by reason of self-abuse ... degenerate beings who, as regards moral character, are very much what eunuchs are represented to be – cunning, deceitful, liars, selfish – in fact, morally insane' (in Turner, 1988: 166). His remedy for such moral insanity was uncompromising – 'the sooner he sinks to his degraded rest the better for himself, and the better for the world which is well rid of him'. Elaine Showalter (in Turner, 1988: 172) summarized Maudsley as a representative of 'Darwinist, determinist, evolutionist psychiatry, which claimed a new social authority as experts on the laws of heredity and the operations of the mind'. Yet, ironically, it is Maudsley who is credited with giving expression to new ideas on mental illness which were to propel psychiatry out of the asylum and into the community.

From asylum to hospital psychiatry

It was Maudsley's name and money (some £30,000 initially, followed by further generous donations) which facilitated the foundation of the Maudsley Hospital in central London in 1915. He insisted that the new hospital dealt with early and acute cases only; had an outpatient department; took about one-third pauper patients with the rest fee-paying; made provision for teaching and research; and was recognized as a school of the University of London (Jones, 1993). As the hospital was completed during the First World War, its initial function was in the service of treating victims of 'shell-shock'. Martin Stone (1984: 245) notes how 'the monolithic theory of hereditary degeneration upon which Victorian psychiatry had based its social and scientific vision was significantly dented as young men of respectable and proven character were reduced to mental wrecks after a few months in the trenches'. The orthodoxies of asylum-based, biological psychiatry increasingly came under challenge and by the 1920s had lost much credibility. This challenge came primarily from the army doctors who had gained considerable experience in dealing with the 'nervous disorders' of shell-shocked servicemen. Their focus on the environmental causes of mental distress effectively undermined the bio-determinist approaches of the asylum doctors. Although they had little previous experience in dealing with mental disorders they had been open to the influence of the as yet under-utilized theories and techniques of psychology and psychoanalysis. Prior to 1914 there were only a handful of British doctors using psychological methods and they were mainly in private practice. Indeed, the vast majority of British neurologists and asylum doctors were at best disinterested, at worst openly hostile to Freudian ideas (Stone, 1985). By the end of the war this had changed dramatically.

The boom in outpatient facilities after the war (such as those at the Maudsley Hospital and the Tavistock Clinic which opened in 1920) initially began as an attempt to deal with the 100,000 plus ex-servicemen who were suffering from the long-term effects of 'shell-shock'. However, many of the medical doctors involved in experimenting with psychotherapeutic techniques soon began to make a strong contribution to the discourse about mental disorder (Pilgrim and Treacher, 1992). They contributed to the expansion of the British Psychological Society through the development of its Medical Section in 1919 and the British Psychoanalytical Society was formed in the same year. It is generally acknowledged that the influence of 'shell-shock' and the growth of psychological methods in its treatment promoted a transformation in mental health theory and practice. However, although psychological theories opened up a new site of practice for psychiatry in the treatment of acute neurosis *outside* the asylum, very little changed for those considered chronically insane inside the asylums. These people continued to receive primarily physical (usually chemical) treatments in generally poor environments (Bean, 1980). These two strands in the development of psychiatry co-existed rather than conflicted in the inter-war years. The medical psychotherapists worked in private practice or in the 'shell-shock' outpatient clinics whereas the asylum doctors continued to practise hospital-based biological psychiatry. Moreover, although at one level psychological and psychoanalytic theories and practices represented (and continue to represent) an important challenge to the biologically focused psychiatric establishment, the potential threat posed was to a great extent neutralized by their absorption into an overarching medical framework. The medical psychotherapists not only continued to use the language of illness but also to exploit the authority inherent in their medical status. A dynamic of change had been set in motion from outside of the profession, but this resulted in a new and permanent eclecticism rather than internal conflict (Pilgrim and Treacher, 1992).

The front-line approach to the treatment of mental disorder taken by the 'shell-shock' doctors emphasized the importance of voluntary relationships and contributed to a climate of change towards the liberalization of the lunacy laws to facilitate such voluntary treatment. In 1924, the Royal Commission on Lunacy and Mental Disorder (the Macmillan Commission) was set up in response to allegations of neglect and brutality brought against the staff of Prestwich Hospital by Dr Montagu Lomax, a doctor who had worked as a locum at Prestwich during the First World War. Although Lomax's observations were fiercely disputed at the time, his insights prompted the Macmillan Commission to enquire into the whole legal and administrative system governing the certification, confinement and treatment of those of unsound mind in England and Wales. In particular, attention focused on whether provision should be made for treatment without certification. The Commission's ideas on the nature of mental distress, treatment and after-care, and its use of medical terminology were highly significant and influential. It proposed a holistic approach to mental and physical illness, recognizing that the distinction between the two was on the whole an arbitrary exercise. Thus there were calls for an interactive and complementary approach between general and psychological medicine. The move towards voluntarism was apparent in the Commission's contradiction of the Poor Law principle of deterrence. There was a clear commitment to the principle of prevention demonstrated in the call for early intervention and treatment without certification. Certification was to be a last resort. There were recommendations that local authorities should develop outpatient clinics, provide psychiatric beds in general hospitals and psychiatric after-care services. Indeed, the medical terminology adopted throughout the inquiry signalled an important break with the past. No longer would there be references to 'asylums', 'attendants' and 'lunatics', but 'hospitals', 'nurses' and 'patients' (Jones, 1993).

The conclusions and recommendations of the Macmillan Commission formed the basis of the 1930 *Mental Treatment Act*. This Act gave full legislative support to the introduction of voluntary treatment and outpatient facilities, and, some have argued, signalled the consolidation of medical hegemony in the field of mental distress (Pilgrim and Rogers, 1993; Rogers and Pilgrim, 1996). The legalism of the 1890 *Lunacy Act* which had sought to regulate the coercive aspects of psychiatry such as confinement, forcible treatment and restraint, was replaced by a medicalism which played down these elements making them 'a matter of clinical judgment rather than a subject for legal regulation' (Fennell, 1996: 10). Under the Act, the Board of Control (which replaced the Lunacy Commission) 'became a willing ally in the profession's desire to promote the view of psychiatry as fit to take its place in mainstream medicine' (Fennell, 1996: 280). The Board was remodelled as a medically dominated body, actively promoting experimentation with physical treatments. Professional training in psychiatry was by now well established with the more senior posts in mental hospitals restricted to those medical practitioners possessing the Diploma in Psychological Medicine or the Diploma in Mental Diseases. Similarly, formal training for psychiatric social workers and occupational therapists emerged during this period, contributing to the overall therapeutic orientation and endorsement of the 'illness' model.

Clearly, the legal sanctioning of voluntary relationships under the 1930 *Mental Treatment Act* was an important element in facilitating the transfer from a custodial to a therapeutic ethos in psychiatric theory and practice. Additionally, there was a desire to promote mental health as a public health issue. The Feversham Committee of 1939 identified the need for a programme of mental health education. However, this did not get off the ground until after the Second World War. During the war, plans for social reconstruction were drawn up which included mental health services in the overall plan for a new National Health Service. The Report, *The Future Organisation of the Psychiatric Services* (1945) was co-authored by the Royal Medico-Psychological Association, the British Medical Association and the Royal College of Physicians. It concluded that 'there is everything to be said for making the administrative structure of psychiatry exactly the same in principle and even in major detail as that of other branches of medicine' (in Jones, 1993: 143), hence consolidating and going beyond the findings of the earlier Macmillan Commission.

From hospital to community psychiatry

During the second half of the twentieth century, the large mental hospital increasingly ceased to be seen as the ideal environment for treating the mentally ill. The number of residents in the asylums peaked at around 150,000 in 1955, but by 1992 this figure had plummeted to just 50,000. The trend towards de-institutionalization and care in the community was signalled in the *Report of the 1954–7 Royal Commission on the Law relating to Mental Illness and Mental Deficiency* (the *Percy Report*). The Commission's brief was not only to return to the vexed question of compulsory detention of the mentally ill, but also to examine the organizational and administrative structures governing the provision of services outside the hospital setting. The integration of mental health services into the new National Health Service was proving to be more problematic than anticipated. The Commission extended the arguments of the earlier Macmillan Commission regarding certification insofar as it unequivocally identified mental disorder as *illness* and recommended further relaxation of the legal barriers to early treatment. Although legal detention was not completely abandoned the Commission recommended that all matters relating to admission and discharge, whether 'formal' or 'informal', were to be governed by the medical profession. Rogers and Pilgrim (1996: 69) argue that the Commission based its recommendations on a number of assumptions that it accepted uncritically. First, that mental illness was something that could be reliably identified by psychiatrists. Second, that once mental illness was identified, this automatically implied a *need* for treatment. Third, that early treatment was so crucial that it justified the loss of liberty. Fourth, that psychiatric treatment was effective, and finally that the integrity of medics was beyond doubt.

In relation to the provision of services in the community the Commission not only endorsed the development of local services, but also indicated a preference for community over hospital care. However, the aspirations of the Percy Commission towards community care were not given full legislative support in the subsequent *Mental Health Act* of 1959. Local authorities were *invited*, not required, to produce community care plans, and since no additional money was made available to facilitate such developments, in the short term progress tended to be patchy. Nevertheless, the numbers of patients in mental hospitals continued to decline as the consensus of support for community care grew. Moreover, the policy of discharge accelerated in the early 1960s when, following a keynote speech by the then Health Minister, Enoch Powell, at MIND's annual conference in 1961, plans were put forward to further reduce and eventually phase out the old mental hospitals altogether. The 1962 *Hospital Plan for England and Wales* proposed the development of small-scale psychiatric units in District General Hospitals and it was envisaged that local authorities would provide a full range of domiciliary services to support patients in their own homes. The decision to relocate mainstream psychiatric practice in the District General Hospitals clearly reinforced the medical approach to the care and treatment of the mentally distressed, ironically at a time when social models of care were demonstrating some success (as, for example, in the therapeutic communities established by Bion, Jones, Main and others in the post-war period). In this sense, such far-reaching change in policy direction warrants careful consideration. Indeed it has prompted numerous commentators to speculate as to the primary motivating force(s) underpinning the process of change.

The drug revolution

It is popularly believed that it was the development of major tranquillizing drugs in the 1950s that enabled the movement of massive numbers of mental patients into the community. However, although the major tranquillizers were introduced in 1954, their use was not widespread until much later (Busfield, 1986). Prior (1993) argues that patients were being transferred to the community up to ten years before major tranquillizers were introduced. Scull (1977: 83) suggests that while the introduction of the major tranquillizers may have facilitated the *management* of mental patients discharged into the community, they were not responsible for the policy itself. He concludes that falling numbers were a 'continuation rather than a departure from pre-existing trends'. Moreover, the pharmacological argument fails to explain why it was that community care policies were applied generically to institutional populations of children, older people and the mentally disabled, and not just to the mentally ill.

Therapeutic optimism

While Whig versions of psychiatric history have long asserted that it was the drug revolution which enabled the doors of the asylums to be opened and the process of de-institutionalization to begin, this interpretation has been challenged by those who argue that there were significant developments dating back to the 1930s and 1940s which contributed to a mood of therapeutic optimism. Nolan (1993: 98) notes how, during this period, psychiatry found itself travelling along two paths – 'just as it was beginning to espouse a social model of care in the community, it was also pursuing with unequalled vigour new "medical treatments" in the hospitals'. During the inter-war years there had been a resurgence in Victorian bio-determinism, a period characterized as an age of experimentation (Fennell, 1996). Clearly the 1930 *Mental Treatment Act* had begun to generate a new spirit of medico-scientific progress. Although controversial, the introduction of the new physical treatments from the late 1930s onwards (insulin coma therapy, electroconvulsive therapy and psychosurgery) fostered a belief that a technological solution to the problem of mental illness was imminent.

Alongside (although in stark contrast to) the new biological approaches, the psychoanalytically orientated army psychiatrists once more led the way in pioneering new approaches to mental distress. This was clearly facilitated by the appointment of the Director of the Tavistock Clinic as head of the Army Psychiatric Services in 1939, along with two other colleagues. Rather than adopting an individualized approach to traumatized servicemen, these clinicians experimented with group methods, emphasizing the role of the social environment in aiding recovery. Such an approach demanded fundamental change in the organization and management of the hospital structure to make it more flexible and egalitarian. 'Therapeutic communities' were developed by Tom Main, Maxwell Jones and others during the Second World War and the model was subsequently transported into the civilian setting where the same pioneers set about unlocking the doors of the traditional mental hospitals in an effort to humanize the care and treatment of the institutionalized insane (see Chapter 3). By the 1950s most hospitals had open-door policies. It has been argued, therefore, that it was this wave of post-war innovation and optimism that facilitated the transformation from institution-based to community-based mental health care (Busfield, 1986).

Fiscal crisis

Scull's (1977: 1) preferred explanation for what he terms the 'state sponsored policy of closing down asylums' is an economic one. He argues that the social control mechanism of segregation which epitomized nineteenth century approaches to managing the mad became increasingly costly to the state and could not be sustained in the context of the emergence of welfarism in the post-Second World War era. He suggests that there was not so much a shift in policy direction from hospital to community care but from 'segregation in the asylum to neglect in the community' (Busfield, 1986: 328). However, Busfield notes that Scull's account of 'decarceration' is also historically inaccurate. The 'fiscal crisis of the state' was not a phenomenon of the 1950s (a time of relative prosperity and economic growth) but rather emerged in the 1970s. Moreover, Scull's account fails to acknowledge the complexities surrounding patterns of expenditure on mental health services during this period, in particular the significance of the expansion of primary mental health services. Busfield highlights the reorientation of resources away from chronic long-term patients towards acute services dealing with less serious mental health problems. Therefore, while overall expenditure increased, this was at the expense of the more chronically mentally ill. Thus, while Scull makes salient criticisms of the subsequent failure to guarantee the provision of adequate and appropriate services for the mentally ill, either in hospital or in the community, his economic arguments cannot account for the introduction of the policy in the first instance.

Anti-institutional critiques

Increasingly from the 1950s onwards there emerged both within and outside of the psychiatric profession a growing body of critical work that reflected a profound disenchantment with institutional care in all of its forms. Jones (1993) refers to these as the 'ideologies of destruction'. Writings on the sociology of deviance had developed out of the work of Lemert and Mead of the Chicago School in the early 1950s. Together with phenomenology, ethnomethodology, labelling theory and symbolic interactionism, these perspectives informed the development of a powerful critical literature around the nature, causes and responses to mental illness. Goffman's ideas on *The Characteristics of Total Institutions* (1957) and *The Moral Career of the Mental Patient* (1959) pointed to the dehumanizing effects of psychiatric institutions on their inmates. At the Tavistock Clinic, R. D. Laing had published *The Divided Self* (1959) in which he questioned the nature of mental illness and the validity of psychiatric diagnosis. Meanwhile, the right-wing libertarian psychiatrist Thomas Szasz was asserting *The Myth of Mental Illness* (1961) and accusing his colleagues of tyranny.

It was not only social critics or dissident clinicians who attacked institutional psychiatry. The social psychiatrists, such as Russell Barton, George Brown and John Wing, although they were still located within the mainstream of psychiatric theory and practice, spoke out against the anti-therapeutic nature of institutional life. Barton's work, *Institutional Neurosis* (1959), heavily influenced by his experiences of working with survivors of the Nazi concentration camps, demonstrated the severe negative effects of long-term institutionalization. Studies by Brown (1959), Wing and Freudenberg (1961) and Brown and Wing (1962) all confirmed the same pattern of social withdrawal and apathy in long-stay patients. This wave of negative criticism was intensified by the subsequent publication of a number of official inquiries into neglect and ill-treatment in various hospitals from 1969 onwards (Beardshaw, 1981; Martin, 1984). These served to confirm the pessimism both within and outside of the profession as to whether it was possible to reform the psychiatric hospitals. Nevertheless, Prior (1993) questions the suggestion that the anti-institutional critiques precipitated the policy of community care, arguing that they only gained momentum after the trend towards de-institutionalization had already begun.

Changing professional ideologies

Rather than look for causal factors to account for the policy of de-institutionalization others have sought to contextualize the process in terms of evolutionary ideas within the knowledge base of psychiatry itself. In particular, 'the psychiatrization of new problems and the differentiation of the psychiatric population' have been considered significant (Rose, 1986: 83). As more and more categories of 'disorder' have been identified, codified and classified, so greater numbers of people have come under the clinical gaze of psychiatry. Busfield (1986: 342) has noted the significance of 'changes in the content of therapeutic ideas about the causes and treatment of mental disorders'. She points to the redirection of therapeutic activity away from the environment (as in moral treatment) towards the individual. This was clearly facilitated by the influence of Freudian ideas about neurosis and the rising popularity of psychotherapeutic techniques in the clinical setting. Coupled with the expansion of state medical and social services the institutional setting became less significant and no longer represented the ideal location for psychiatric practice. Prior (1991) develops this point further in his observation that the process of change in psychiatric theory, policy and practice throughout the twentieth century has to be understood in the context of particular views of madness and organizational arrangements. For example, as long as the focus of psychiatry was on degeneracy theory, it was necessary to pursue a policy of institutional segregation and control. However, the broadening out of models of madness, particularly under the influence of psychology and psychoanalysis, demanded an organizational structure that was compatible with and facilitated voluntary therapeutic relationships between 'client' and 'therapist'.

While there is disagreement as to what precipitated the drive towards community care policy it is nevertheless clear that a professional and political consensus in favour of de-institutionalization existed in the post-war era. However, the history of its implementation is characterized by slow and uneven progress. Anxieties were increasingly expressed regarding an apparent over-riding concern to run down and close the long-stay hospitals without the provision of adequate alternative services in the community.

From care *in* the community to care *by* the community

By the 1970s the old mental hospitals were decaying due to lack of investment while the extent and adequacy of some of the local authority community services was being called into question. The lack of legislative powers to compel local authorities to provide services was recognized as a serious barrier to pursuing community care. The limitations to progress were reflected in the tone of official documents. The 1975 White Paper, *Better Services for the Mentally Ill* was a key document setting out the framework for the development of a national policy on mental health. Hunter (1992: 172) cites its four broad policy objectives:

1   The expansion of local authority personal social services to provide residential, domiciliary, day care and social work support.
2   The relocation of specialist services in local settings.
3   The establishment of the right organizational links.
4   A significant improvement in staffing.

However, despite such recognition of what needed to be done, pessimism remained about the ability to fulfil these objectives. Financial pressures started to undermine community care policy further with central government imposing stringent controls over public expenditure. The early optimism concerning the possibility of rehabilitating the chronically mentally ill was proving to be unfounded and it was increasingly recognized that there was a residual group of 'new' long-stay patients. Additionally, although there was considerable criticism of the old hospital system from within psychiatry itself, and some psychiatrists were keen to develop new sites of practice in the community, nevertheless it was clear that others were reluctant to make the break (Davidge *et al.*, 1993; Rogers and Pilgrim, 1996).

By the late 1970s it was evident that the state's interpretation of community care was changing. In the broader context of fiscal crisis and economic recession the new Conservative Government of 1979 demonstrated an increasing antagonism towards the public administration model of welfare which had been characteristic of the postwar period. The apparent political and professional consensus that existed around the need for publicly provided services *in* the community was shattered and instead the emphasis shifted towards care *by* the community. Furthermore, feminist analyses began to highlight the fact that it is women who carry primary responsibility for caring in these contexts (Finch and Groves, 1983; Wilson, 1977). Throughout the early 1980s the Government pursued a low-key 'hands-off' approach, giving little more than rhetorical support for community care. In 1983 it announced its *Care in the Community Initiative* which enabled health authorities to transfer funds to local authorities and voluntary bodies to pay for services for those moving from hospitals to the community. However, despite decades of discussion around the need for effective collaboration on the provision of services, the health authorities and the local social services authorities were generally very slow to embrace joint initiatives. By the mid-1980s there was a veritable pot-pourri of provision with no systematic planning or resourcing. In the main, however, it was the hospital model of provision that still dominated. This has led some commentators to suggest that what was happening was not so much a process of de-institutionalization but *re-institutionalization* (Busfield, 1986; Rogers and Pilgrim, 1996).

Although there was another major review of mental health legislation between 1978 and 1982, there was scant attention paid to the issue of poor service provision and standards of mental health care. The new *Mental Health Act* of 1983 was primarily concerned with the extremely important, but nevertheless relatively narrow, long-standing issue of the civil liberties of detained patients. The broader problems surrounding the provision of adequate and effective mental health services were left unaddressed. The House of Commons Social Services Committee (*The Short Report*) was highly critical of the Government's apathy:

> The stage has now been reached where the rhetoric of community care has to be matched by action ... our analysis and the evidence we have heard led us to believe that the Department is not in every respect living up to its duties of central management.
>
> (1985, para 27)

In 1986, the Audit Commission reported critically on local government and the health authorities. In particular it highlighted the persisting role confusion between the two in the provision of community care and the slow progress being made towards the 1975 White Paper targets. It was heavily critical of the enormous mismatch between resources and need. Although some 80–90 per cent of people with mental health problems were now living in the community, more than 80 per cent of available resources were being spent in the hospital sector.

Realizing that some action had to be taken the Government appointed Sir Roy Griffiths to produce recommendations for the future of community care. Drawing on the conclusions of the *Short Report* and the Audit Commission, the *Griffiths Report* (1988) re-affirmed the criticisms concerning inadequate resourcing of community care policy and the abdication of responsibility by central government. Nevertheless, Griffiths' broader suggestions regarding the reorganization of health and welfare services were in line with the Government's enthusiasm for a mixed economy of welfare, involving a combination of statutory, voluntary and private sector provision. Unsurprisingly, it was this aspect of the *Griffiths Report* that the Government chose to accentuate and the criticisms were played down. Griffiths recommended that in order to reduce the role confusion between agencies, local authority social service departments:

- should be given the lead role in the provision of community care;
- should receive cash limited funds;
- should undertake 'needs-led' assessments and design individual 'packages of care';
- should become 'enabling agencies', purchasing and overseeing care, NOT directly providing it.

Griffiths' proposals were enshrined in the 1989 White Paper *Caring for People* (DoH, 1989) and the subsequent *National Health Service and Community Care Act* of 1990. This legislation brought about unprecedented generic structural changes in the delivery of health and welfare services. The Act introduced a market-oriented approach to the provision of health and welfare services in general via such mechanisms as compulsory competitive tendering; the creation of the purchaser–provider split; the encouragement of general practitioner fund-holding and self-governing hospital trusts; and the drive towards quantitative measures of services and outputs (Le Grand and Bartlett, 1993). This has been referred to as the 'commodification' of welfare services (Offe, 1984).

While the sentiments of the new legislation (such as the promotion of consumer choice and greater independence) were greeted with widespread support, the means by which community care was to be achieved (through wholesale upheaval of health and welfare services) soon attracted fierce criticism. Evaluative research post-implementation has reinforced the suspicion that the changes owe more to ideology than to reason (Ballard, 1994; Grant, 1995; Hadley and Clough, 1997; Henwood, 1994; Lewis *et al.*, 1995; Marchant, 1995; NHSCA, 1995; NISW, 1995). These studies point to a series of fundamental contradictions in the legislation, which have led to confusion and alienation for both service users and providers alongside frustration and demoralization at declining standards of service.

In the context of mental health service provision, community care for people in mental distress is based on the premise that needs-led assessments will lead to the provision of appropriate services. However, in order for needs-led assessments to work there has to be effective co-operation between the various health and social care professionals involved and sufficient resources to meet those needs. While the rhetoric of government ministers focused on a commitment to giving people who use mental health services more of a say, the reality highlighted a system plagued by gross under-funding and role confusion. Moreover, by early 1994 the debate around community care rapidly became entangled in a series of moral panics surrounding a small number of high profile cases. These include the case of Ben Silcock who climbed into the lion enclosure at London Zoo, and the killing of Jonathan Zito by Christopher Clunis at a London Underground station. The moral dilemma of either protecting the public or preserving the civil and human rights of those in mental distress is by no means new. However, the intensity of the media response to these and similar cases fed into a series of knee-jerk reactions by government in an effort to allay public anxieties. These included the introduction (as of 1 April 1994) of Supervision Registers to identify and provide information on service users 'who are, or are liable to be, at risk of committing serious violence or suicide, or of serious self neglect' (NHS Management Executive, 1994a: 1) and the introduction of the *Mental Health (Patients in the Community) Act 1995* which (as of 1 April 1996) made provision for the supervised discharge of mentally ill people in the community. Both of these developments are at odds with the philosophies of empowerment and social integration. The legitimacy of such coercive measures has been challenged through research and the findings of official inquiry reports which have pointed the finger squarely at structural failures in the system (see, for example, Audit Commission, 1994; Blom-Cooper *et al.*, 1995; DoH, 1996; 1994a; 1994b; House of Commons Health Select Committee, 1994; Mental Health Foundation, 1994; Nuffield Provincial Hospitals Trust, 1994; Ritchie *et al.*, 1994; Sheppard, 1995). (See also Chapter 6 for a fuller discussion of crises of legitimacy in mental health services.)

Taylor (1994/95: 85) observes that 'to relocate someone geographically and physically within 'the community' as opposed to the mental hospital does not automatically lead to integration with that community'. Research by Prior (1993) revealed that although their physical environment had changed and the organizational pattern of service delivery had changed, there was little change on the social networks of the patients in his study one year after discharge. This leads Taylor (1994/95: 81) to conclude that 'while community care policies are designed to integrate people with mental illnesses into the community those same policies also act to isolate them from that community'. Indeed, he suggests that this confirms Bott's (1975) argument that there is a basic conflict between the mentally distressed person and society – whereby he or she is positioned as 'other' or 'inferior' – and that this alienation is likely to reassert itself whatever form mental health services may take. Consequently, it can be considered naïve to promote community care without first tackling the historical tendency to abuse, neglect and limit the opportunities of mentally distressed people (O'Hagan, 1993).

Medicalization and social control

Treacher and Baruch (1981: 120) contend that although during the course of the twentieth century the British mental health system became more complex, 'there remains a striking uniformity in the way that the majority of patients are processed by the system'. This appears to indicate that while the organizational base of psychiatry has moved from the asylum to the community, the ideological base has changed very little (Pilgrim, 1993). For most of the twentieth century it was the medical model that dominated mental health theory and practice. Ingleby argues that the achievement of a visible link with mainstream medicine has been crucially significant for the professional development of psychiatry:

> Psychiatry's leaders have always been sensible enough to see that without this link the profession's power would be disastrously reduced: though non-physical approaches can be assimilated as long as they satisfy positivistic criteria, the link with medicine provides the essential lifeline of respectability and trust.
>
> (1983: 165)

Such commentators are keen to emphasize the social control functions of psychiatry through the medicalization of madness. The ability to categorize certain behaviours as 'illnesses' is considered an extremely powerful tool as it enables the psychiatrist to invalidate a person's actions and achieve social control through the application of a medical label (Ewins, 1974). In particular, the power of medical explanations of mental distress lies in the potential to divest a person's behaviour of any political significance, rendering their actions meaningless 'symptoms' which can only be deciphered by the expert psychiatrist (Treacher and Baruch, 1981).

Ronald Leifer (1990: 250) argues that 'redefining deviance as mental illness requires a covering ideology to justify what otherwise would be seen as the unconstitutional confinement of innocent persons. The medical model of psychiatry serves as such an ideology'. The medical model shifts explanations of human behaviour from an essentially moral framework of meaning (where it is assumed individuals have free choice and responsibility for their actions in relation to the judgment of law or social convention) to an illness framework (where the failure or refusal to conform is seen as a consequence of biochemical, social or psychological disturbance). Leifer (1990: 250) argues, 'this switch in semantics promotes a transformation of perceptions which converts the person labelled as mentally ill into the kind of object upon which psychiatrists represent themselves as qualified to act'. He suggests that the medical model is well suited as an ideology since not only does it draw its authority and legitimacy from 'science', but from a branch of science that is 'benevolent' and 'compassionate' – medicine.

Although the cornerstone of the medical model of mental health is that there is an organic basis to mental distress, many variations of the basic illness model have evolved within psychiatry. Indeed, with the incorporation of psychological and psychoanalytic approaches from the early part of the twentieth century, psychiatry became more therapeutically eclectic. This trend continued throughout the century with explanatory frameworks and therapeutic practices increasing in complexity and sophistication (for a fuller discussion of alternative models of therapeutic intervention see Chapter 3). Clare notes:

> The medical model, in short, takes into account not merely the symptoms, syndrome, or disease but the person who suffers, his personal and social situation, his biological, psychological, and social status.
>
> (in Treacher and Baruch, 1981: 122)

Some commentators have argued that it is through this apparent tolerance of other positions and frameworks that psychiatry has strengthened its professional position (Baruch and Treacher, 1978; Busfield, 1986; Ramon, 1985). Goldie (in Treacher and Baruch, 1981) has suggested that it is precisely because psychiatry adheres to an eclectic approach that it is able to absorb any potential challenge to its authority. This chameleon-like quality is also noted by Fennell (1996: 278) who observes that 'historically, periods of major psychotherapeutic change have coincided with attempts to remake the image of psychiatry and psychiatrists'. In this sense Treacher and Baruch (1981) suggest that the medical model operates as a powerful smokescreen disguising the hegemony of the psychiatric profession.

Additionally, the therapeutic discourse of medicine provides a more covert, extra-legal form of social control. This underpins the observation in Pilgrim and Rogers (1993) that psychiatry's practices have become less blatantly associated with coercive social control. Following Foucault (1977), a number of commentators have argued how increasingly during the twentieth century the exercise of power and control over the masses relied less on direct bodily sanction and incarceration and more on surveillance and monitoring under the benevolent gaze of 'disciplinary networks' of health and welfare professionals (Donzelot, 1980; Rose, 1979, 1985, 1989, 1990). Although each profession has developed within its own distinct institutional framework, professional practices have converged at the site of discourse and knowledge derived from within 'the psy complex'

(Rose, 1985). So powerful are these ideas that it is argued individuals have become 'self-regulating', assessing and passing judgement on their own psychological health against 'norms' of 'appropriate' behaviour:

> Manifold conceptions percolate through society as to what a person of a specific age and gender and of a specific social position should want and what he or she should be capable of. If the person is willing but unable to function, the search for disease begins.
>
> (De Swaan, 1990: 23)

De Swaan argues that the medical model or 'regime' is now so firmly established that it can be applied with more flexibility and less rigidity. He says that we live under a 'light medical regime', 'not so much healthy as not-yet-sick' (1990: 57). This indicates a process of medicalization of everyday life to the extent that people have become 'proto-patients' – in a state of constant watchfulness for *potential* illness long before any actual distress or discomfort; and 'proto-professionals' – experts 'in redefining everyday troubles as problems amenable to treatment by this or that profession' (1990: 14). That is, the tendency in Western societies to interpret ever more social and emotional difficulties within a medical, particularly psychiatric, framework reflects the rising expectation that all human problems should be amenable to solution through the services of a 'professional' (Zola, 1972).

> The total medical regime operates within a wider society that has been increasingly medicalized and in which a medical regime in a lighter form has expanded further and further.
>
> (De Swaan, 1990: 56)

However, De Swaan warns against naïve ways of conceiving of doctors as 'all powerful'. While he acknowledges medical dominance, he corrects and confirms a more complicated understanding of power relationships – within and between different groups of professionals in the mental health field, between professionals and the public, and between professionals and patients.

Within and between professionals

It is not just psychiatrists who benefit from the medical model. While psychiatrists have primary responsibility for the care and treatment of the mentally distressed, other professionals compete with them for influence and power. The 'psy-professions' – clinical psychologists, psychotherapists, mental health nurses and mental health social workers – 'all achieved their present standing by exploiting the power inherent in the medical model' (Ingleby, 1983: 164). Williams (1993) suggests that 'mystification' is an important element in this. Professionals promote their services as unique and indispensable. In doing so they create a dependency on their skills and reduce the areas of knowledge and experience they have in common with their clients. This increases the social distance between them. The claim to specialist knowledge is central as the professional's claim to be qualified to advise; to know better than their clients; to be trusted by the public; to be given reward and prestige, all rest on it. However, as De Swaan observes, the various mental health professions are still in the relatively early stages of development. The boundaries around their activities remain flexible and disputed and they are under constant pressure to justify themselves to their own ranks as well as to the outside world by stressing the needs that they fulfil. He notes:

> The establishment of a profession owes much to intellectual achievements – sometimes even to scientific accomplishments – but it is also the result of a struggle with adjacent professionalizing groups for the demarcation of competences between them, and accordingly for access to potential clienteles.
>
> (De Swaan, 1990: 14)

A whole variety of different professions jostle for space, attention and independence in the mental health field. In this sense it could be argued that the psychiatric profession has never commanded an absolutely monopolistic or hegemonic status over the identification and treatment of mental distress, nor indeed has the medical model within the profession itself. Although it has been possible to trace the often burgeoning aspirations of the medical profession in the mental health field, it must be acknowledged that this has not been straightforward. Sedgwick observes:

> Innovation and reform in psychiatry have always been linked with the arrival of certain conditions of political possibility, which have been variously either promoted or blocked by ideological tendencies and social movements.
>
> (1982: 205)

Certainly, there are many examples of ideas and innovations in the mental health field that have gone against the grain of prevailing psychiatric knowledge and practice. For example, the significance of moral treatment and the non-restraint movement in the nineteenth century, the influence of psychology and psychoanalysis during the early decades of the twentieth century and the development of social psychiatry in the post-war period.

Between professionals and the public

There have been various responses to the question of why it is that the general public seems to accept the legitimacy of psychiatry. Some have suggested this might be due to the fact that lay people are so poorly informed about the limitations of psychiatric knowledge and competence (Pilgrim, 1992a). Others suggest that the public has been infantilized into accepting medical authority through a process of socialization (Ingleby, 1983). On the other hand, De Swaan argues that people are happy to hand over responsibility for the management of madness to medical experts as they do not want to accept responsibility for it themselves. As Parker *et al.* state:

> The reason why the medical model has such power now is that people trust medicine and will be willing actively to assist the medical control of the mentally ill.
>
> (1995: 10)

Similarly, it has to be recognized that members of the public often actively seek out the services of psychiatrists and other mental health professionals, suggesting that such relationships are far more consensual than is usually acknowledged. Pilgrim and Rogers (1993: 92) indicate that there exists a 'cultural consensus' between professionals and the public about the management of everyday problems of living. This is not to deny the powerful position of mental health professionals but rather illustrates how 'social regulation occurs by agreement and with actual (or perceived) benefits to the client'. Additionally, medical regimes may be checked and directed through public criticism of the legitimacy of medical power (De Swaan, 1990; see Chapter 6 for a fuller discussion of crises of legitimacy in psychiatry).

Between professionals and patients

De Swaan correctly observes that patients, albeit from a structurally more dependent position, are nonetheless active participants in the interaction between themselves and clinicians. While it is true that clinical research and practice 'has tended either to exclude the views of patients or portray them as the passive objects of study' (Pilgrim and Rogers, 1993: 161), more recently two significant discourses have emerged which have posed a challenge to the dominance of medical authority – those of *'consumerism'* and *'user empowerment'*.

The notion of mental health *'consumer'* or *'service user'* has to be understood in the wider context of the restructuring of health and welfare provision in general during the 1980s and 1990s. The introduction of general management principles has tended to modify the clinical view of services, challenging the dominance of professionals in the design and delivery of health and welfare. The importance of services being accountable to 'the patient' has been emphasized (Griffiths, 1988) along with 'consumer choice', through the development of Quality Assurance mechanisms, the Patient's Charter and a commitment to Customer Care. In the mental health field, it might be argued that these changes appear to indicate a shift away from the medical model and a sensitization to the views of the mentally distressed. However, as Pilgrim and Rogers (1993: 167) suggest, the enduring 'power of professionals to impede or dictate choice renders it problematic'. Moreover, critical research has revealed structural inequalities, with the capacity for making choices being restricted by geographical location, ability to pay, class, gender, race and ethnicity, and age (Ahmad, 1993; Blackburn, 1991; Cornwell, 1984; Kelleher and Hillier, 1996; Nettleton, 1995; Payne, 1991; Torkington, 1983, 1991; Victor, 1991). Although the philosophy of the market is both powerful and persuasive, the allure of consumer choice, efficiency, value for money and quality disguises fundamental tensions and contradictions inherent in the commodification of human distress. Thus, while the valorization of free market principles and economic libertarianism under Thatcherism ironically created a space for the development of 'consumer agendas', closer examination reveals serious obstacles to realizing this potential increase in power and influence for mental health service users (Pilgrim, 1992a).

By contrast the concept of *user empowerment* is firmly rooted in the individual and collective struggles of users of psychiatric services. Although there is a long history of individual resistance to psychiatric oppression, it has been the growing collective activities of mental health users since the 1970s and 1980s which has been of crucial significance in recent times. The mental health users' movement, as with other civil rights movements, developed out of a quest for self-determination, coupled with a fundamental sense of injustice at the way in which medical psychiatry renders mental distress meaningless.

It is informed by the principle that everyone has the right to be taken seriously and have their experiences recognized as meaningful. Crucially this includes the right to own and define one's own distress and to have a decisive influence in finding solutions to that distress (Hopton, 1994/95). Through a process of consciousness-raising, mental health service users have begun to challenge and change attitudes towards mental distress and the provision of mental health care. Some have been keen to emphasize the scope for reforming the system by inviting mental health workers to engage with users of their services in a process of empowerment, arguing that only user-centred services will provide genuine alternatives to the medical model (Wallcraft, 1996). Others have adopted a more radical, separatist stance, choosing not to associate with professionals but developing their own self-help initiatives (O'Hagan, 1993).

Clearly, it is possible to recognize *both* hegemonic *and* oppositional tendencies in the evolution of mental health theory, policy and practice throughout the twentieth century. Prior (1993: 47–48) challenges the notion that changes in the care and management of the mentally ill are the end product of the wishes and activities of any specific individuals or groups either from within or from outside psychiatry. Following Merton, he argues that such a view 'tends to ignore the possibility that innovations in the organization of social life often begin as the result of the unintended consequences of unplanned actions rather than of rationally calculated schemes of activity'. Similarly, Parker *et al.* (1995: 16) emphasize that it is naïve to entertain conspiracy theories of nasty psychiatrists. Rather it is necessary to recognize 'a historical process that positions psychiatrists, clinical psychologists and other mental health professionals in relations of power over "users" or "consumers" of services'.

Modern psychiatry is no longer (if indeed it ever was) monolithic (Rose, 1986). The sites for its practice have proliferated in terms of its geography (from asylums/mental hospitals to general hospitals to community); classification (the differentiation of 'new' problems); and 'techniques of normalization' (new therapies, new markets, new distribution of professional powers). The chapter which follows turns to an exploration of the most influential alternative contributions to mental health theory and practice that have emerged from outside psychiatry.

3 Alternative models of managing mental distress

By the mid-nineteenth century asylum doctors had convinced the medical profession that they had developed a new medical specialism of psychiatry, and the government of the day had effectively granted psychiatrists total control of public sector mental health services (Scull, 1993). Furthermore, all mental health legislation from the *1890 Lunacy Act* through to the *1983 Mental Health Act* reaffirms the primacy of the medical profession within statutory mental health services. Although many psychiatrists adopt an eclectic approach to mental health care, their authority comes from the fact that they are medical doctors. As all psychiatrists complete basic medical and surgical training before specializing in psychiatry, this has inevitably led to the predominance of the medical model of mental illness/mental distress within the National Health Service. Thus most users of mental health services are given a clinical diagnosis (which defines, categorizes and labels their distress as if it were an infection or a physical malfunction), and are likely to be prescribed medication as the principal (or even the only) treatment for their 'condition'.

The aforementioned eclecticism of some psychiatrists and the 'prehistory' of medical psychiatry make it difficult to determine what constitutes a true alternative to medical psychiatry. For example, Thomas Withers, William Battie and Nathaniel Cotton, the eighteenth century British pioneers of a psychiatry based on the primacy of interpersonal relationships and social therapy, were physicians who happened to specialize in the treatment of mental illness (Nolan, 1993). On the Continent there is a long tradition of medical doctors using psychological approaches to the treatment of mental distress. This can be traced back through Alfred Adler (1870–1937), Carl Jung (1875–1961), Pierre Janet (1859–1947) and Sigmund Freud (1856–1939) to Jean-Martin Charcot (1835–1893) and, albeit ambiguously, to Franz Anton Mesmer (1734–1815) (Ellenberger, 1970). Furthermore, notwithstanding the importance of the work of Emil Kraepelin (1856–1926) in developing an eclectic model of psychiatry based on neurology, brain anatomy, experimental psychology and the significance of life events (Ellenberger, 1970), a split remains *within* psychiatry between those who believe strongly in physical causation of mental distress and those who believe that social and emotional factors are of greater significance (see Clare, 1976; Cohen, 1989; Szasz, 1979b). As Diana Gittins observes in her detailed history of Severalls Hospital in Essex, such contradictions have often been evident in the tension between the prescriptions of social policy on mental health and contemporary practice in mental health care (Gittins, 1998a).

The situation is further complicated by the fact that many psychiatrists who have moved away from biological/medical models of understanding mental distress, and even in some cases developed systems of therapy which may be learnt and practised by non-physicians, have themselves continued to practise as medical psychiatrists. Such figures include not only Janet, Adler and Jung; but also late twentieth century psychiatrists such as Maxwell Jones and Tom Main (pioneers of therapeutic communities), Eric Berne (founder of transactional analysis), R. D. Laing and David Cooper (the so-called anti-psychiatrists) and even biological psychiatry's most outspoken critic Thomas Szasz (who has remained a professor of psychiatry).

It is therefore less confusing if psychotherapeutic approaches which may be studied and practised by those who have received no formal medical training are described as complementary to psychiatry rather than as alternatives to psychiatry. This terminology would seem to be appropriate because, although such therapies may be practised outside mainstream psychiatry as alternative therapies, a thorough search of relevant indexes and abstracts will almost certainly reveal that there is someone somewhere offering such therapies within mainstream mental health services. Furthermore, many people who undergo psychoanalysis, psychotherapy and counselling do not have major mental health problems or serious emotional difficulties. Rather, they willingly undergo therapy in search of personal growth and/or enlightenment as to the significance of their innermost thoughts and feelings.

However, there are literally hundreds of such approaches, some of which are not widely known to the general public (for example, Internal Family Systems – see Goulding and Schwartz, 1995); and some of which have, at one time or another, been quite fashionable and popular. As the main focus of this book is the development of a critical analysis of psychiatry itself, we will address this problem by discussing some of those models of psychotherapy which may be practised by professionals other than psychiatrists, but which have nevertheless had an impact on mainstream mental health services. The most important therapeutic approaches in this respect have been psychoanalysis, behavioural psychology and the phenomenological counselling/psychotherapy developed by Carl Rogers. As David Pilgrim (1997) has noted, attempts to make a distinction between counselling and psychotherapy are fraught with difficulty. Therefore we will use the two terms interchangeably.

Psychoanalysis

Of all the alternatives to medical psychiatry, psychoanalysis has the most ambiguous relationship with the psychiatric establishment. Although some authorities argue that the term should be applied only to the theories of Freud, the term is used here in its broader application to refer to those theories which build directly on the work of Freud, Adler and Jung – including the various factions of the British School of Psychoanalysis (see Fordham, 1966; Kohon, 1986). The common theme to all these approaches is that the client (or analysand) explores experiences (especially early childhood experiences) and emotions through developing a relationship with his/her analyst. As this relationship develops, the client supposedly achieves clearer insight into how s/he behaves in relationships with others, so that the analyst may help him/her to understand and change responses that are causing problems in his/her interpersonal relationships.

The ambiguous relationship between medical psychiatry and psychoanalysis arises not only from the fact that Freud, Jung and Adler were themselves medical doctors who specialized in psychiatry, but also from the enduring influence which psychoanalysis had on many of psychiatry's innovators throughout the twentieth century. In the British context, many psychiatrists have undergone psychoanalytic training while working at the Tavistock Clinic (Mullan, 1995; Nolan, 1993). Many medically trained psychiatrists have been associated with the Tavistock Clinic and have been innovators in mental heath care. Some of these include: John Bowlby, the authority on child care and developmental psychology; Tom Main, who developed the principles of the therapeutic community at Northfield Military Hospital and the Cassel Hospital; D. W. Winnicott, the leading child psychiatrist; and R. D. Laing, who was a prominent figure in the anti-psychiatry movement of the 1960s and 1970s (Jones, 1993; Mullan, 1995).

However, the influence of psychoanalysis on British psychiatry extends beyond those people who have been associated with the Tavistock Clinic. For example, psychoanalytical concepts have often been either a prominent feature, or at least a sub-text to standard textbooks on psychiatry (see Batchelor, 1969; Sim, 1981). David Clark (who pioneered the application of the therapeutic community approach to large long-stay psychiatric hospitals) underwent psychoanalysis and trained in group and individual psychotherapy at the Maudsley Hospital before moving to Fulbourn (Clark, 1996). Also, whereas psychoanalysis is usually associated with the treatment of neurotic symptoms (Cohn, 1997), some psychiatrists who have completed psychoanalytic training have successfully applied the principles of psychoanalysis to the care of psychotic individuals (for example, Berke *et al.*, 1995; Conran, 1986).

Despite these influences, however, psychoanalysis in its purest form has not made a great impact on mainstream psychiatric services. There are several inter-related reasons for this. First, it takes several years of personal analysis, academic study and clinical training for a person to train as a psychoanalyst. Inevitably this is expensive, and relatively few psychiatrists have the time, energy and financial means to undergo such training after already spending several years training to be a doctor. Second, possibly because of the financial implications, few other mental health professionals undertake training in psycho-analysis. Indeed, psychoanalytical concepts have rarely been discussed in any depth in British textbooks of mental health nursing, and mental health nurses almost certainly represent the largest single group of professionals working with people with mental distress. Admittedly, social work has had brief flirtations with psychoanalysis, but there are relatively few books which address the relevance of psychoanalysis to social work in any depth, and the psychoanalytical approach is generally regarded as having too narrow a focus to be useful in most social work contexts (Coulshed, 1988).

Although the influence of psychoanalysis on mainstream mental health services is not without significance, it is by no means wide-spread, and psychoanalysis proper is rarely available through the National Health Service. At the most basic level, psychoanalysis is closely related to psychiatry in that the early pioneers of psychoanaly-sis were psychiatrists who were not content to merely identify symptoms but sought to establish the meaning of symptoms in the context of each individual patient's life circumstances (Freud, 1953). In this sense psychoanalysis is not so much a challenge to medical psychiatry as complementary to it. Thus psychiatrists may study psychoanalysis alongside medicine without encountering any major theoretical conflicts and contradictions. In the British context, psychoanalytically trained psychiatrists were at the forefront of developing therapeutic communities for the care and treatment of mentally distressed individuals. The therapeutic community movement began in military hospitals during the Second World War and maintained an influence on institutional psychiatry until the 1970s. Despite the continued existence of a small number of such units this approach has now been unfashionable for many years, although there is now renewed interest in therapeutic communities as a treatment modality for people with personality disorders (Campling and Haigh, 1999). The main historical significance of the therapeutic community movement, though, is that therapeutic communities in NHS psychiatric hospitals played an important role in challenging authoritarian attitudes amongst traditional psychiatric hospital staff. This prepared the ground for later developments in democratic mental health care (Clark, 1974; Pilgrim, 1997).

Inasmuch as psychoanalysis may be studied and practised by individuals with no prior medical training, it may be considered to be an alternative model of managing mental distress as well as an intervention complementary to more orthodox methods of psychiatric intervention. However, although there are a small number of psychoanalytically orientated psychotherapy services within the NHS, psychoanalysis is more usually offered by therapists in private practice. As it is a form of therapy that is both intense and long term, psychoanalysis is costly in terms of both time and money. It is therefore mainly people who are prepared to make great sacrifices or who have relatively high incomes who choose to undergo psychoanalysis (Farrell, 1991). On the other hand, psychoanalytical ideas have captured the imagination of various intellectuals, screenwriters, playwrights and authors, and have therefore been exposed to a wide audience. In this sense the influence which psychoanalytical thought has had on lay concepts of mental health and mental distress cannot be overlooked.

Behavioural psychology

Whereas psychoanalysis originates from a tradition of dynamic psychiatry within medicine, the origins of behavioural psychology lay within the separate intellectual tradition of experimental psychology (Lanyon and Lanyon, 1978; Nicolson, 1998). One of its greatest champions, B. F. Skinner, successfully applied the principles of behavioural psychology in a variety of educational and training contexts. During the 1970s and 1980s behavioural therapy (also known as behaviour modification and operant conditioning) was very much in vogue in mental health services and services for people with learning difficulties. Behavioural therapy is based on the presupposition that patterns of behaviour such as phobic reactions, severe anxiety, lack of volition and anti-social habits are learnt behaviours which can be eradicated and replaced with more constructive and more socially acceptable behaviours. During the 1970s and 1980s these principles were often applied with enthusiasm. Articles were published describing how behavioural therapy had been used successfully to treat severe psychiatric conditions such as elective mutism, obsessive-compulsive rituals, 'disruptive behaviour' and the effects of institutionalization (Andrews, 1988; Clayton, 1981; Fraser *et al.*, 1981; Hall and Rosenthal, 1973; Zikis, 1983).

Nevertheless, behavioural therapy has always been a controversial form of treatment; so much so that a document outlining ethical guidelines for its use was once published for the (British) National Health Service (HMSO, 1980). The crux of the ethical dilemmas around the use of behavioural therapy is that it is based on the conditioning of operant behaviour. Operant behaviour may be defined as behaviour which is both observable and susceptible to voluntary control, and the fundamental premise of operant conditioning is that behaviours which are rewarded will become more frequent while behaviours which are not rewarded will become less frequent. Accordingly, therapists seek to control clients' environments and manipulate the consequences of clients' behaviours in order to eliminate some behaviours and encourage others. It is this potential for therapists to dominate and control clients which has informed the critique of behavioural therapy (Capra, 1983); although at least one critic of behaviourism has acknowledged that it may be 'a valuable tool for the promotion of certain types of learning' (Rogers, 1980: 55).

B. F. Skinner (1973, 1974) mounted a robust defence of the ethics of behavioural therapy against the many criticisms which have been levelled at it. Nevertheless, criticism of operant conditioning continued and, in the context of mental health services, it has now been largely displaced by cognitive behavioural psychotherapy (see Salkovskis, 1993). However, although there are situations where the language of behavioural therapy has been used to justify cruel interventions (such as the 'control units' that were established at Wakefield Prison and Wormwood Scrubs during the 1970s; see Ackroyd *et al.*, 1980), it is important to put these into perspective.

Skinner consistently argued that reward is usually more effective than punishment, while, in the context of the National Health Service, the authorities issued clear ethical guidelines for would-be behavioural therapists (HMSO, 1980). However, despite the protestations of Skinner and the publication of ethical guidelines, the displacement of operant conditioning by cognitive behavioural approaches probably owes as much to a growing perception of operant conditioning as crude, mechanistic, punitive and readily open to abuse as it does to research-based evidence of the effectiveness of cognitive therapy (Masson, 1990; Parker *et al.*, 1995).

The clinical founders of cognitive therapy, Albert Ellis and Aaron Beck, first developed this form of therapy in the 1960s but it was not until the 1970s that the significance of their ideas was widely acknowledged within psychiatry and clinical psychology (Beck, 1967; Ellis, 1962; Pilgrim, 1997). Cognitive-behavioural therapy is similar to operant conditioning in the sense that practitioners plan therapeutic intervention by considering the relationship between antecedents, behaviours and consequences. However, cognitive-behavioural therapists have less direct control over their clients than practitioners of behaviour modification. Rather, they help their clients to understand the relationship between antecedents, irrational thoughts and emotions, maladaptive behaviour and the consequences of such behaviour. They then teach coping strategies to their clients which might also be applicable to other behavioural and emotional conflicts, and therefore have the potential to foster independence from, rather than dependence on, the therapist (Trower *et al.*, 1988).

In the heavily managerialized National Health Service of the 1990s, cognitive-behavioural therapy has some advantages over other modes of intervention. First, there is strong clinical evidence that it is an effective form of treatment (Haddock and Slade, 1996). Second, as cognitive-behavioural therapy is neither manipulative nor involves in-depth exploration of emotional turmoil, its techniques may be safely utilized by mental health workers who are not themselves formally qualified clinical psychologists or psychoanalysts/psychotherapists (Parker *et al.*, 1995). Third, in many cases, only a relatively short period of therapy will be needed, so it is relatively inexpensive (Trower *et al.*, 1988). However, Parker *et al.* point out that cognitive-behavioural therapy is also firmly located within a positivist tradition and suggest that it might not necessarily be compatible with philosophies of care which emphasize respect for diversity rather than the promotion of 'conformity' and the policing of 'normality'. Similarly, while recognizing the attractiveness of cognitive-behavioural therapy to cost-conscious NHS managers, Richard House (1996) questions whether cognitive-behavioural therapists can respond effectively to a person's psychic pain.

While there is clear evidence of the efficacy of behavioural and cognitive-behavioural therapies, cognitive-behavioural therapy is essentially prescriptive. This makes it difficult to reconcile such approaches with the other major psychotherapeutic 'discovery' of the late twentieth century: person-centred psychotherapy.

Rogerian person-centred counselling and psychotherapy

Carl Rogers first articulated his theory of personality and person-centred psychotherapy (originally called client-centred therapy) in the late 1940s and early 1950s. Rogers' theory of personality and psychotherapy is really quite complex (see Rogers, 1951). However, in summary, Rogers argues that all human beings have a need to realize their full intellectual, emotional and creative potential. In order to realize this potential they need to be regarded positively by others or they will experience dissonance between their image of themselves and the image of themselves reflected back to them by others. Where such dissonance occurs, a person will protect his/her self-image by adopting negative feelings towards others and/or developing an unrealistic view of his/her own abilities and personality traits. In Rogerian therapy the therapist establishes an accepting, unconditional relationship so that the client may re-evaluate negative feelings about themselves and others feelings, without feeling threatened.

Although Rogers published his definitive work on client-centred therapy in 1951, it did not really begin to make an impact on public mental health services in the UK until the late 1970s/early 1980s. There is no obvious explanation for why such a long time elapsed before it made an impact or why it became fashionable when it did. However, there are several factors which may have contributed to the delay in its emergence into mainstream discourses of mental health in Britain.

The Second World War gave rise to a uniquely British liberalizing movement within British psychiatry in the form of the therapeutic community movement. This was spearheaded by psychiatrists such as Tom Main who had worked at the Northfield military hospital and Maxwell Jones who had worked at the Mill Hill military hospital while serving in the Royal Army Medical Corps during the Second World War. At both Northfield and Mill Hill, new approaches to mental health care were developed based on the principle of discussing problems of daily living in groups. After the war, Jones founded the Henderson Hospital, while from 1946 until 1976 Main was the director of the Cassel Hospital. These became two of the best-known therapeutic communities in British mental health services. Together with Russell Barton's work on rehabilitation and institutionalization at Severalls Hospital and David Clark's further development of the theory and practice of the therapeutic community approach at Fulbourn Hospital in Cambridge, they represented the spearhead of a liberal and progressive tendency which existed within mainstream British psychiatry from the Second World War until the mid-1970s. For example, Russell Barton's (1959) *Institutional Neurosis* had a profound impact on the training and education of British mental health nurses throughout the 1960s and 1970s; David Clark's (1974) *Social Therapy in Psychiatry* was published as a Penguin paperback which is still to be found in many professional libraries; while Tom Main and Maxwell Jones both made significant contributions to the literature on therapeutic communities. Alongside these very influential psychiatrists there were many others who made similar contributions to advances in social psychiatry during this period. These include Bertram Mandelbrote at Littlemore Hospital, T. P. Rees at Warlingham Park Hospital, Duncan Macmillan at Mapperley Hospital, Francis Pilkington at Moorhaven Hospital and many others (Clark, 1996).

Another progressive tendency which overlapped with the therapeutic community/social psychiatry developments, both temporally and conceptually, was the anti-psychiatry movement. Although some writers include Thomas Szasz in discussions of anti-psychiatry, the anti-psychiatrists 'proper' were self-styled existentialists, while Szasz has always preferred to be described as a libertarian psychiatrist. Moreover, Szasz's political analysis of mental health overlaps only slightly with the British-based anti-psychiatrists critique of coercion in psychiatry (see Clare, 1976). The appropriateness of the term anti-psychiatry has subsequently been contested by many of those to whom the label has been applied. The term is used here to refer to that group of psychiatrists who were involved with the Philadelphia Association, a group of intellectuals which was founded in the early 1960s and who sought to understand mental distress through existentialist philosophy and psychoanalytical theory. The Philadelphia Association included several psychiatrists including David Cooper, R. D. Laing, Joseph Berke, Morton Schatzman, Loren Mosher and John Heaton. R. D. Laing was unquestionably the best-known member of the Philadelphia Association, although David Cooper was the author of four books which were widely read at the time, while Joseph Berke and Morton Schatzman also wrote important books which reflected the outlook of the Philadelphia Association. Laing had begun to articulate his ideas about mental health in the late 1950s. Although he continued to write until the time of his death in 1989, his last significant work on mental health was published in 1982, while Cooper's last major book was published in 1980, six years before his death in 1986 (Cooper, 1980; Laing, A., 1994; Laing, R. D., 1959, 1982). By the mid-1970s anti-psychiatry was no longer the *cause célèbre* that it had once been amongst Britain's left-wing and *avant-garde* intelligentsia (Clark, 1974; Laing, A., 1994; Mullan, 1995). Indeed, left-wing politics was itself no longer fashionable – a development underlined by the eighteen-year period of Conservative rule which began in 1979. The decline of anti-psychiatry in the mid-1970s to early 1980s coincided with two inter-related developments. First, many of the main protagonists of social psychiatry were approaching retirement age. Second, as mental health policy became increasingly orientated towards community care, interest in the therapeutic community movement began to wane. Indeed, its pioneering work had to some extent been overshadowed by the anti-psychiatrists' own attempts at developing therapeutic communities at Villa 21 in Shenley Hospital and Kingsley Hall in Central London, as well as later in the various houses run by the Philadelphia and Arbours Associations (Berke *et al.*, 1995; Cooper *et al.*, 1989). (There is a fuller discussion of the significance of anti-psychiatry in Chapter 4.)

The demise of anti-psychiatry and the retirement of many of the social psychiatrists who were the stalwarts of the therapeutic community movement coincided with the exposure of neglect and mistreatment at several British psychiatric and learning disabilities hospitals (Beardshaw, 1981; Martin, 1984). As this crisis within mental health services emerged at a time when no further innovations were evident within British mental health care, it is perhaps not surprising that Rogerian person-centred therapy now came into vogue (Cooper and Lewis, 1995; Hopton, 1997a). Rogerian therapy was now well established and respected on the other side of the Atlantic, its founder claimed that it was inherently anti-oppressive, and through the development of a 'New Age' personal growth movement it was becoming the new psychotherapeutic fad amongst the intelligentsia (Capra, 1983; Rogers, 1980). However, as Masson (1990) has observed, while Rogerian person-centred therapy is a relatively benign intervention, it is rarely of any help to people experiencing severe mental distress or to those compulsorily detained in mental health institutions. For example, persons who are deeply depressed or who are experiencing psychotic thought disorder may not benefit from Rogerian counselling because they are unable to keep their thoughts clearly focused on their problems. More importantly, where people are compulsorily detained in hospital, it is nothing less than hypocrisy for a nurse, social worker or therapist to encourage a person to believe that s/he has all the resources necessary to solve their problems when a consultant psychiatrist has near absolute power over decisions about home leave and discharge from hospital.

Other alternative strategies for managing mental distress

There are so many different systems of psychotherapy, and even different schools of thought regarding the same approach to psychotherapy (Pilgrim, 1997), that it is not possible to evaluate the relevance of each separate school of thought to the continuing advancement of knowledge about mental health and mental distress. Nevertheless, there are at least two systems of psychotherapy which, by virtue of their broader appeal, merit some specific mention: Transactional Analysis and Gestalt Therapy.

Gestalt Therapy usually occurs in the context of a group or work-shop and is primarily concerned with helping people become 'whole' by completing 'unfinished business' and confronting their innermost feelings. Typically this is achieved through role-plays, where people are encouraged to 'act out' what they are feeling in the here and now, and the double chair technique where a person acts out a conversation between different parts of his/her own psyche, changing chairs to signify which part of his/her self is speaking at a particular moment.

Transactional Analysis is also somewhat 'gimmicky' and often practised in group contexts, however it is more like other psycho-therapies than is Gestalt Therapy. Transactional Analysis includes both a theory of personality based on a study of ego-states, and a system of psychotherapy based on the analysis of transactions (i.e. interactions between individuals) that occur in treatment sessions. There are three ego-states: Parent, Adult and Child (sometimes described collectively as the PAC model). However, 'Parent' may be sub-divided into 'Critical Parent' and 'Nurturing Parent', while 'Child' may be sub-divided into 'Free Child' and 'Adapted Child'. These ego-states are conceptually similar but not synonymous with the Freudian concepts of Superego, Ego and Id. Specifically, 'Parent' refers to ideas about appropriate ways to think and behave which have been uncritically copied from parents and other authority figures. 'Adult' refers to all rational thought and attempts to evaluate ideas and information objectively. 'Free Child' refers to freely expressing emotions and/or gratifying desires without regard to societal pressures. 'Adapted Child' refers to censoring emotions and desires in accordance with societal pressures. The basic theory of Transactional Analysis is that conversations (transactions) may be analysed by considering which ego-state a person is sending a message from; which ego-state s/he expects the recipient of the message to respond from; which ego-state the recipient of the message replies from and which ego-state the recipient of the original instigator of the interaction responds from. Other important concepts in Transactional Analysis include the concept of a 'Game' (a series of transactions in which one person has something to gain by giving mixed messages and anyone else involved will end up feeling confused, misunderstood, exploited or resentful), and the concept of a 'Life Script' (an unconscious life plan formulated in childhood and reinforced by parents, 'confirmed' and 'justified' by subsequent life events and culminating in a chosen alternative).

Transactional Analysis is important because its originator, Eric Berne, always made it clear that he intended to develop a populist model of interpersonal psychology and psychotherapy; an objective that was realized when books on Transactional Analysis by himself and others became best-sellers (Berne, 1968; Harris, 1973). Transactional Analysis has drifted in and out of fashion with mental health professionals and members of other caring professions since the late 1960s. However, despite a peak in interest in the mid-1970s, it has failed to have a substantial impact on mental health care policy and practice in the UK (Stewart and Joines, 1987).

Whereas Eric Berne sought to articulate sophisticated theoretical ideas using jargon based on everyday language (rather than on obscure Latin phrases or scientific terminology), Fritz Perls (the originator of Gestalt Therapy) and his followers openly admitted that their approach to psychotherapy was not an intellectual one. Many of its protagonists have shown a marked reluctance to discuss the theoretical basis of Gestalt Therapy in any depth and instead emphasize the importance of learning about Gestalt Therapy through simply experiencing it (Houston, 1982; Stevens, 1975). They argue that the important thing is to be open to new experiences that occur in therapy, rather than to endlessly talk about one's anxieties and 'hang-ups'. While this is an unusual approach, it is not unique. Neo-

Vygotskian therapy and therapeutic communities of various types are also based on the principle that simply talking about one's mental health problems is inadequate (see Kennard and Roberts, 1983; Newman and Holzman, 1993). However, they differ from Gestalt Therapy inasmuch as advocates of these approaches usually have no problems about putting forward intellectual arguments about their method to encourage people to partake of therapy. In contrast to this, many Gestalt therapists would argue that experience must come first and theorizing can follow. However, like Rogerian therapy and Transactional Analysis, Gestalt Therapy has enjoyed periods of great popularity amongst devotees of the personal growth movement (Capra, 1983) as well as with self-styled liberal and radical mental health professionals.

Since the 1980s and 1990s, the now somewhat vaguely defined concept of 'counselling' or 'therapy' has increasingly become a feature of media discussions of unfortunate events or perceived sources of stress (see, for example, Braid, 1995; Grant, 1992; Pilgrim, 1997). However, the newsletter cum catalogue of one of Britain's most prominent suppliers of books on psychotherapy (The Anglo-American Book Company in Carmarthen) is now dominated by books and adverts for expensive seminars and training courses on 'Neuro-Linguistic Programming' (NLP). NLP is a therapeutic approach which was developed in the USA during the late 1970s and early 1980s by John Grinder and Richard Bandler. It is a collection of techniques for changing one's own behaviour and the behaviour of others. Those who promote, market and practise NLP often describe it using such terms as 'practical', 'observation-based', and 'the study of subjective experience' and refer to models, presuppositions and techniques. However, although NLP incorporates elements of hypnosis and behavioural psychology, its presuppositions (which are listed on many NLP-related Internet sites; e.g. Cox, 1996; Kirby, 1997) read more like homespun philosophy than scientific precepts. NLP is marketed as being useful to salespeople and educators as well as therapists, and combines techniques borrowed from cognitive therapy, Gestalt Therapy and hypnotherapy (Bandler and Grinder, 1982; Cox, 1996; Grinder and Bandler, 1981). It is unashamedly populist, openly appealing to 'common sense' pragmatism, and antipathetic to ideologies of mental health which seem to promote the mystification of mental health problems. At the same time it is conceded that most of the evidence for its efficacy is anecdotal (Bandler and Grinder, 1982; Kirby, 1997). However, while some studies have questioned some of the claims made for NLP (for example, Von Bergen *et al.*,

1997), there is (albeit limited) evidence from practitioners of NLP that some of its techniques may be helpful to certain people in certain circumstances (Curreen, 1996; Stanton, 1996).

It is difficult to assess the extent to which the rise in popularity of these newer and less 'scientific' alternative/complementary therapies for mental distress were an inspiration to the growth in self-help groups for people with mental distress, and/or to organized resistance to the power and authority of statutory mental health services. However, it is interesting to note that the mental health service users' movement (at least in the British context) did not begin to have much influence on how mental health services were organized and delivered until the mid-1980s. This was precisely when these various 'new' ideologies of mental health had become a significant aspect of popular culture and were frequently evident in all aspects of media representation. Nevertheless, it is important to remember that critiques of mental health services by service users have always been a feature of mental health services (Campbell, 1991; Clark, 1974). There are other cultural developments which might explain why providers of mental health services began to take more notice of service users in the 1980s. For example, the so-called anti-psychiatry of the 1960s and 1970s (which will be reviewed in the next chapter) had directly challenged the legitimacy of psychiatry *from within* at a time when challenges to the social, political and cultural *status quo* were not uncommon (Cooper, 1968). Therefore, it is possible that people who entered the mental health professions at that time might have continued to be more receptive to criticism than their predecessors as they rose to more senior positions within their professions. Also, although anti-psychiatry and the counterculture of which it was part were largely spent forces by the mid-1970s, a more reserved approach to promoting the right of users of public services to choice and freedom from paternalism was a key feature of the New Right politics of the Conservative governments between 1979 and 1997 (Clarke and Newman, 1997; Pilgrim and Rogers, 1993).

Self-help groups and the mental health service users' movement

Notwithstanding the long tradition of service users writing critically about mental health services, one of the defining characteristics of the occupational cultures of many mental health professions until the mid-1980s was a tendency to dismiss the grievances of such writers as either arising from a presumed psychopathology or politically motivated anger (Campbell, 1989; Lindow, 1993; Rogers and Pilgrim, 1991). Thus, immediately prior to the foundation of Survivors Speak Out and MINDlink, *circa* 1986, there were two distinct groupings of organizations representing the views of users of mental health services. On one side, there were radical organizations such as the Campaign Against Psychiatric Oppression which was explicitly anti-professional and advocated avoiding all contact with statutory mental health services. On the other were organizations such as MIND and the National Schizophrenia Fellowship, whose members included many mental health professionals as well as service users and their relatives. These organizations sought (and continue to seek) to reform existing mental health services and make them more sensitive to the needs of people who experience mental distress, whether those needs were defined by service users, their relatives or carers, or by mental health professionals.

In 1986, the foundation of Survivors Speak Out, a support network for individual service users, represented the beginning of a new era for users' organizations in which criticism of existing mental health services and self-determination for service users ceased to be marginal issues. The formation of Survivors Speak Out led indirectly to the formation of MINDlink (an organization exclusively for past and present service users under the umbrella of MIND, Britain's oldest, biggest and most influential organization campaigning for better mental health services) and the UK Advocacy Network (UKAN). People associated with these organizations have subsequently played important roles in developing organizations such as the Hearing Voices Network and the National Self-Harm Network which provide practical advice and support to service users but also campaign for more user-centred services. The fact that most policy-makers now consider it to be good practice to include representatives of mental health service users' organizations on any working parties, committees or commissions concerned with mental health issues stands as testimony to how successful these organizations have been (Hopton, 1997a).

On balance, these developments are to be welcomed. Users' organizations are involved both in shaping mainstream services to render them more sensitive to the needs of service users, and in providing alternatives for those who remain reluctant to use the mainstream services. However, this shift in professional attitudes towards service users has brought new problems. As one of us has commented elsewhere (Hopton, 1997b; Hopton and Glenister, 1996), the approach to service user representation tends to smack of tokenism, and there is little recognition that mental health service users are not a homogeneous group. Consequently, little attention has been paid to the question of 'empowering' individual service users in their day-to-day contact with individual mental health professionals. There is a very real risk that statutory mental health services will slip back into an increasingly repressive role as the Government reaffirms its commitment to ideologies which demand that mentally distressed persons must be 'controlled' as well as cared for (Pilgrim and Rogers, 1998).

An alternative perspective on the current state of affairs concerning user involvement has been put forward by Andy Smith, who styles himself a survivor of mental health services. In his view, because funders will finance service provision but not campaigning, some users' groups have opted to concentrate on their advice and support functions and have become service providers. He has suggested that this may be detrimental to users' organizations in two ways. First, funders may see this as a cheap option and may not finance user-led initiatives adequately. Second, he feels that this may mute campaigning activity as user organizations may feel that they have to be diplomatic so as to keep their source of funding intact (Smith, 1998).

Overlaps and tensions between different approaches to therapy

It is important not to underestimate the contribution of the mental health service users' movement to the development of mental health services which are more sensitive to the needs of people with mental distress. Even so, many of the ideas about care that it promotes have been around for some time in one form or another. Certainly, the writings of service users about how to manage self-harm and hearing voices have challenged many of psychiatry's assumptions and presumptions about such phenomena, but Jung and Laing also believed that psychotic experiences could be rendered intelligible and might in some cases be beneficial. Similarly, there are certain cultural contexts where self-harm is not necessarily considered to be a pathological behaviour (for example, tattooing, body-piercing, ornamental branding and scarification) (Weinberg, 1995).

Furthermore, the premise on which much of the writing of service users is based is that people who have had personal experience of traumatic events and/or mental distress can be more helpful to people experiencing mental distress than highly qualified professionals (Lindow, 1990; Pembroke, 1994). In fact, this is an idea which has been around since at least the end of the Second World War, when some people who had been incarcerated in Nazi concentration camps drew on their experiences of surviving the Holocaust/Shoah to develop new psychotherapeutic approaches. For example, Bruno Bettelheim and Viktor Frankl, who had both been practising psychoanalysts prior to their incarceration, used their psychoanalytical training to make sense of their predicament, and subsequently used their experiences to develop radically new approaches to psychotherapy (Bettelheim, 1986; Frankl, 1984). Similarly, Eugene Heimler (who trained as a psychiatric social worker *after* his incarceration in Auschwitz and other concentration camps) drew on his experiences as a concentration camp survivor and political refugee to develop an innovative approach to working with mentally distressed unemployed people in West London (Heimler, 1967). The main significance of Heimler's work in this respect is that he found that the knowledge and skills he had acquired in his (then) psychoanalytically orientated social work training had not prepared him for working with people who had effectively been labelled 'unemployable'. Faced with this dilemma, he reflected on his own experiences of surviving the Holocaust, facing political turmoil in his native Hungary and emigrating to Britain to identify what had enabled him to overcome these difficulties. From this he developed a different style of therapeutic intervention based on these insights (Heimler, 1962).

However, it is not only the mental health service users' movement which has 'reinvented the wheel'. Within mainstream psychiatry itself, there have been several historical junctures when certain prominent psychiatrists have focused on mental distress as human experience to be transcended, rather than as illness to be cured. For example, this was implicit in aspects of the approach adopted by Battie and Withers in the early eighteenth century; the philosophy of care at the York Retreat was based on such principles; while the therapeutic communities and anti-psychiatry of the late twentieth century are based on a psychosocial model of mental distress. It is difficult to assess how far the pioneers of each of these new approaches to managing mental distress were consciously influenced by their predecessors. However, to the extent that they were, this has seldom been understood by their followers and imitators. Consequently, a recurring theme in the literature about mental health promotion and mental health care has been the claim that each innovation is heralded as a truly radical idea: a claim that does not always stand up to critical analysis.

This is also noticeable in literature about psychotherapy and social psychology. Here, the similarity between what purport to be quite different approaches to the understanding of the management of mental distress can be remarkable. For example, Gestalt therapists (who emphasize the importance of experiential learning) and practitioners of Transactional Analysis (whose practice is based on elaborate theoretical frameworks) may use many of the same therapeutic techniques (James and Jongeward, 1971; Stewart and Joines, 1987). Similarly practitioners of NLP, despite their claims to be offering something radically different from other therapies, are highly eclectic – borrowing techniques and concepts from hypnotherapy, Gestalt Therapy, operant conditioning, cognitive therapy and humanistic psychology without paying too much attention to the theoretical contradictions which might arise from such indiscriminate eclecticism. Even the pragmatic skills-based model of counselling developed by Gerard Egan uses concepts and techniques which also occur in Rogerian person-centred counselling and cognitive-behavioural therapy (Egan, 1994).

In a sense, it is unfair to single out particular therapeutic approaches and point out what they have borrowed from elsewhere. The reality is that there are more similarities than differences between most of the (non-medical) therapeutic models currently practised. Furthermore, in most cases, those who have developed and popularized the various models have claimed that they have a wider application than the alleviation of mental distress and the promotion of mental health. Carl Rogers applied his ideas to education and even went so far as to imply that the wholesale acceptance of his philosophy might lead to the evolution of a more caring society (Rogers, 1980). Transactional Analysis and NLP have both been adopted by management consultants and educationalists, and – as is the case with Rogerian therapy and psychoanalysis – they have been used to help people seeking personal development as well as to help people overcome emotional, psychological and relationship difficulties. Thus, while the anti-psychiatrists and Thomas Szasz were anxious about the potential for a coercive state to use psychiatry to police dissent, psychiatrization of society is actually occurring through private individuals and organizations freely choosing to invest in the expertise of psychotherapists and counsellors.

It is not our intention to deny that any of the various approaches to therapy has made a significant contribution to our understanding of mental distress and how to manage it. A thorough reading of several issues of MIND's bi-monthly journal *Openmind* will soon reveal that there is plenty of anecdotal and research evidence to suggest that any established approach to mental health care will have both supporters and detractors amongst both mental health professionals and mental health service users. However, there are two problems concerning those therapists who make spurious claims to originality and radical innovation. The first is that it discourages mental health professionals from learning from the past successes and failures of mental health care. The second is that it seduces them into a futile search for *the* great therapeutic approach. Instead of focusing on how to alleviate the effects of the 'here and now', some mental health professionals expend great amounts of time, energy and money seeking the ideal therapeutic intervention – like medieval knights seeking the Holy Grail. For example, conversations with people at any counselling/ psychotherapy seminar or on any counselling/psychotherapy course, will almost certainly lead to the discovery of those who seem to spend their whole life practising therapy, learning new therapeutic techniques, participating in encounter groups and/or undergoing therapy. Similarly, many mental health professionals build up a 'rag-bag' repertoire of interventions from which they can mix and match responses to service users' problems. Such eclecticism may lead to the adoption of a pragmatic approach to therapy which might benefit social users. However, there is also a risk that it will lead to a poor understanding of theoretical considerations such as whether there are any circumstances in which a particular mode of intervention might be contra-indicated.

Together, the incorporation of alternative/complementary models of counselling and psychotherapy into mainstream psychiatry, the overlap between apparently competing approaches to therapy, and the widespread acceptance of the legitimacy of therapeutic ideologies throughout the private and semi-private spheres (e.g. family, sexual relationships, churches, community and voluntary organizations), suggest that concern about mental health is a near-universal trait amongst human beings. Furthermore, the interchange of ideas and techniques between different approaches to mental health promotion, personal development and the management of mental distress would seem to suggest that there can be no single answer to resolve these problems of human existence. One way in which mental health workers may deal with this situation is to assume a post-modernist perspective and simply accept the importance of difference and the richness of diversity. However, the long history of abuse of vulnerable individuals by people who see themselves as specialists in mental health and/or psychotherapy demands that ideologies of mental health and technologies of psychotherapeutic intervention be subjected to critical analysis. In the following chapter, some of the most important critiques of mental health care and psychotherapy will be examined in some detail.

4 Anti-psychiatry
Passing fad or force for change?

Whereas most forms of psychotherapy and social psychiatry exist either alongside or within mainstream psychiatry, there are other therapeutic philosophies which directly challenge its core assumptions. Some of these ideologies, such as Scientology, are quasi-mystical creeds which have very little in common with even the more *avant garde* schools of psychotherapy. The impact of such cults on mainstream concepts of mental distress and mental health is negligible. Others, such as the existentialist psychiatry of R. D. Laing and his associates in the Philadelphia Association and the libertarian psychiatry of Thomas Szasz, have influenced opinions about mental health issues amongst mental health professionals, mental health service users and sections of the intelligentsia. Unlike the founders of 'therapy cults' like Scientology, who are usually lay people, these critics are more likely to be psychiatrists, psychotherapists or psychologists with concerns about the power of psychiatrists and the lack of autonomy of users of mental health services.

As R. D. Laing and Thomas Szasz are perhaps the two most influential critical psychiatrists, the following discussion will focus mainly on their work. Significantly, they developed their critiques during the late 1950s and early 1960s, at around the same time that academics such as Erving Goffman and Michel Foucault were developing their own critiques of psychiatry and mental health services. It was also a time which marked the beginning of an era of rapid and extensive social and political change: the beginning of space exploration, the construction of the Berlin Wall, the emergence of new styles of art, music and fashion. Thus, it would be a mistake to discuss these ground-breaking critiques of psychiatry and mental health services without considering their relationship to other newly developing intellectual ideas and wider social change.

Laing, Cooper and the Philadelphia Association

For a short while during the 1960s and early 1970s Ronald David Laing (alias R. D. Laing or Ronnie Laing) was famous – first in Britain, and later also in America. From 1965 until the early 1970s he appeared on television programmes, published articles in periodicals such as *New Left Review* and was even the subject of a lengthy article in the prestigious American magazine, *Life*. To some sections of the intelligentsia he was almost as much an icon of the so-called counter-culture as more famous figures like Che Guevara, Malcolm X, the Maharishi Mahesh Yogi and The Beatles (Crossley, 1998). Indeed, in the early 1970s Laing undertook a lecture tour in the USA which was arranged by a team that included members of the management team of The Who rock group, and delivered lectures to comparatively large paying audiences (Kotowicz, 1997; Laing, 1994). However, although this period represented the height of Laing's fame, he had made all his significant contributions to our understanding of mental distress before the end of the 1960s (Kotowicz, 1997).

In his first book, *The Divided Self* (Laing, 1959), Laing uses real case studies to illustrate his argument that schizophrenia is comprehensible and that it is possible to establish meaningful communication with a psychotically disturbed person. This was a truly groundbreaking and compassionate text written at a time when the dispassionate clinical descriptions of schizophrenia in most psychiatric textbooks often resembled characterizations in gothic horror films. The following passages are typical of what was being written in psychiatric textbooks until the 1970s:

> Delusions of a bizarre or fantastic nature occur and such patients frequently show a silly fatuous manner, their behaviours being foolish, erratic and accompanied by mannerisms and strange antics.
>
> (Ackner, 1964: 146)

> The following is an illustrative case of [hebephrenic schizophrenia]. The very rapid deterioration to a condition of silly, impulsive activity, with inadequate and inappropriate emotional manifestations, great incoherence of speech and thought, hallucinations and apparently absurd ideas, e.g. of influence ..., is very well shown.
>
> (Batchelor, 1969: 274)

The tone of these passages contrasts sharply with the tone of the following passage from *The Divided Self* which is typical of Laing's approach:

A further attempt to experience real alive feelings may be made by subjecting oneself to intense pain or terror. Thus, one schizophrenic woman who was in the habit of stubbing out her cigarettes on the back of her hand, pressing her thumbs hard against her eyeballs, tearing out her hair, etc., explained that she did such things in order to experience something 'real' ... Hoelderlin once wrote: 'O thou, daughter of the ether, appear to me from your father's gardens and if you may not promise me mortal happiness, then frighten, O frighten my heart with something else.' However, these attempts cannot come to anything.

(Laing, 1965: 145/146)

Unlike some of Laing's later writing, such as his poetry, his personal writings and the rather odd 'stream of consciousness' style of *Bird of Paradise* (Laing, 1967), *The Divided Self* is simultaneously scholarly, radical and thought-provoking. Certainly, all these qualities are evident in some of Laing's later writing. However, for a man who was sceptical of the relevance of 'scientific' approaches to the understanding of mental distress, he seemed to have a poor understanding of what constitutes good qualitative research methodology. For example, in *Sanity, Madness and the Family* (which, like *The Divided Self* was an enlightening and compassionate account of schizophrenic experience) no clear rationale is given for choosing to focus only on female patients (Laing and Esterson, 1964). Furthermore, there was no systematic evaluation of the work at Kingsley Hall, although Berke and Schatzman both wrote about aspects of their work there (Kennard, 1998), while Laing published one paper about what was happening at Kingsley Hall in a French journal in 1968 and gave a very brief account of his work there in one of his later books (Kotowicz, 1997).

While Laing had intellectual interests beyond psychiatry and psychoanalysis and was clearly very knowledgeable, he had a tendency to refer to the works of other great writers without exploring their ideas in any depth. For example, although Laing and others associated with the Philadelphia Association cite existentialist philosophy as an important influence (Laing, 1965; Oakley, 1989), it has been suggested that Laing's own ideas are only loosely connected to existentialism (Kotowicz, 1997). Similarly, in a paper entitled 'The Mystification of Experience', Laing makes a passing reference to the anti-colonialist writings of fellow psychiatrist Frantz Fanon (Laing, 1967: 49–64). Yet nowhere in Laing's writing does he explore the similarity between his own ideas about mental health and those of

Fanon (who, like Laing, had been influenced by psychoanalytical theory and Jean Paul Sartre's existentialism).

Depending on which account you read, the Philadelphia Association was formed late in 1964 or early in 1965 – more or less the same time that the Pelican edition of *The Divided Self* was about to be published. The seven founder members were: R. D. Laing (by then a practising psychoanalyst as well as a psychiatrist), Aaron Esterson, David Cooper (both psychiatrists), Sidney Briskin (a social worker), Raymond Blake (a psychotherapist and group analyst), Joan Cunnold (an artist and former psychiatric nurse) and Clancy Sigal (a writer and political activist) (Cooper *et al.*, 1989; Laing, A., 1994). The Philadelphia Association was set up to pioneer new approaches to mental health care and to acquire and manage premises wherein such approaches might be practised (Mullan, 1995). Although most members of the Philadelphia Association later expressed distaste for the label, Cooper called these approaches 'anti-psychiatry', and the name stuck (Cooper, 1970). The Association acquired a five-year lease on Kingsley Hall, a property in East London, and in June 1965 several members moved in there to establish a therapeutic community. Although therapeutic communities had existed before, Kingsley Hall was different inasmuch as it was more permissive than other therapeutic communities, and its therapeutic philosophy was based on a fusion of psychoanalysis, existentialism and phenomenology (Cooper *et al.*, 1989), rather than on a fusion of social psychiatry and psychoanalysis (Kennard, 1998). Its uniqueness led to visits from intellectuals from other fields (such as the arts) as well as from other psychiatrists. All of these people were keen to learn more about this experiment, and some (for example, Loren Mosher, Joe Berke, John Heaton, Haya Oakley, Chris Oakley, David Goldblatt, Paul Zeal, Morton Schatzman) stayed and became more closely involved with the work of the Philadelphia Association. The playwright David Mercer, who was an occasional visitor to Kingsley Hall, based his play *In Two Minds* on the ideas of Laing and Cooper. He later collaborated with the director Ken Loach on the 1971 film version of this play, *Family Life*, which introduced the ideas of Laing and Cooper to a wider audience (Laing, A., 1994; Mullan, 1995). Although Laing acted as an adviser during the making of *Family Life*, the message of the film is more closely based on the ideas of Cooper than the ideas of Laing, which is apparently why he declined to have his name listed on the credits (Mullan, 1995).

Significantly, several of those who were actively involved in the therapeutic activity at Kingsley Hall subsequently established similar projects of their own. Loren Mosher returned home to the USA where he set up communities similar to Kingsley Hall in California, and later in Washington (Lacey, 1995). In 1970, Morton Schatzman and Joe Berke left the Philadelphia Association and established the Arbours Association in London. These projects and the still functioning Philadelphia Association have struggled to survive and/or have evolved into something less radical than Kingsley Hall. Nevertheless, The Philadelphia Association and The Arbours Association continue to provide a viable alternative to traditional approaches to psychiatric care (Berke *et al.*, 1995; Cooper *et al.*, 1989).

It was Laing's involvement with the Kingsley Hall project that led to his transformation from radical psychiatrist to guru of the counter-culture (Laing, A., 1994). Given the centrality of left-wing politics to the counter-culture, it is in some ways strange that Laing, who never adopted a clear political position, should have been accorded such status. Other members of the Philadelphia Association were much more involved with left-wing politics. For example, Joe Berke did much of the administrative work for the 1967 *Congress on the Dialectics of Liberation* and edited a book about the counter-culture (Berke, 1969, 1997), while much of David Cooper's writing about mental health was explicitly political. On the other hand, audio and visual recordings of Laing show that he was an engaging and charismatic public speaker while his talent for writing poetry probably also helped to endear him to young radical intellectuals. In contrast, the recordings of the *Congress on the Dialectics of Liberation* reveal that David Cooper spoke in a slow, monotonous and more or less accentless voice. In other words, despite the revolutionary tone of his writing, Cooper was not equipped to deliver the sort of inspirational talks which enabled Laing to become a minor celebrity of the counter-culture.

At the time when the Philadelphia Association was founded, Cooper was the senior registrar responsible for a therapeutic community at Shenley Hospital: Villa 21. He held that post from 1962 until 1967, and there seems to have been some cross-fertilization of ideas between those involved with Villa 21 and those involved with Kingsley Hall (Lacey, 1983; Laing, 1994; Mullan, 1995). However, Cooper had very little direct involvement with the Kingsley Hall community and, according to Laing, he may never even have visited Kingsley Hall (Mullan, 1994). It is unclear what Cooper was doing between 1967 and 1972, but in 1970 he resigned from the Philadelphia Association because he felt that it was turning into a bourgeois psychotherapy association (Ticktin, 1997).

During 1972 and 1973 Cooper spent some time in Argentina, which he believed to be one of the most psychiatrized nations in the world, and therefore an ideal setting in which to develop anti-psychiatry (Cooper, 1976; Ticktin, 1997). It is clear from Cooper's own writing and from conversations with people who knew him that his personal life was complicated and that he struggled to maintain his own mental health. In *The Language of Madness* (Cooper, 1980), he refers to having experienced an episode of 'madness', while many aspects of his personal life were complicated and his alcoholism was evident to all those who came into close contact with him. Nevertheless, his books represent a unique contribution to critical studies in mental health. He was far more extreme than Laing in his beliefs about the relationship between family dynamics and mental health and, in his books, Cooper argues that sexual enjoyment and mental health are inextricably intertwined. Also, whereas Laing only dabbled in left-wing politics (Laing, 1967; Kotowicz, 1997), Cooper clearly spelt out how he thought that the political situation in Western capitalist countries contributed to the causation of mental distress. While similar ideas had once been expressed by the psychoanalyst Wilhelm Reich (for example, Reich, 1970, 1975b), Cooper's work was unique inasmuch as he made connections between socialist models of understanding mental health and the existentialist therapeutic philosophy of the Philadelphia Association.

Although Laing and Cooper were undoubtedly the leading lights of the British anti-psychiatry movement, they were not the only figures developing new radical approaches to understanding mental distress at this time. In the USA, Loren Mosher and others were also working on radical alternatives to traditional psychiatry and mainstream psychotherapy (Mosher, 1996; Radical Therapist Collective, 1974). In Italy, Franco Basaglia and a group of associates developed innovative democratic approaches to psychiatric care in Gorizia and Trieste, and were instrumental in persuading the Italian government to pass a law phasing out psychiatric hospitals (Kotowicz, 1997; Parker *et al.*, 1995). In West Germany, a psychiatrist named Wolfgang Huber founded the Socialist Patients' Collective of Heidelberg which adopted the position that mental and physical illness were reactions against the misery caused by capitalism, alienation, pollution and repressive sexual morality (Spandler, 1992). The Socialist Patients' Collective of Heidelberg were almost certainly the most explicitly political of all the anti-psychiatry groups of the 1960s and 1970s. After a political struggle with his employers at the University of Heidelberg, which culminated in Huber and some of his patients occupying the clinic,

Huber and several other members of the collective were arrested and imprisoned, apparently because of links they had with the Baader-Meinhof terrorist group (Spandler, 1992, cf. Kotowicz, 1997).

The association of anti-psychiatry with the counter-culture was both its greatest strength and its greatest weakness. The adoption of anti-psychiatry as a *cause célèbre* by intellectuals associated with the counter-culture assured Laing and his colleagues of a platform and a receptive audience. This may even have contributed to psychiatric reform by inspiring young people to enter the mental health professions (Crossley, 1998; Hopton, forthcoming). However, as the counter-culture gradually faded into obscurity, anti-psychiatry came to be seen as just one of many would-be radical ideologies which emerged between the mid-1960s and the mid-1970s. Indeed, despite the value of *The Divided Self* as a plea for a more sympathetic understanding of schizophrenic experience, mainstream psychiatry had always viewed anti-psychiatry as 'a cult with much of the associated mysticism' (Sim, 1981: 585). Unfortunately, notwithstanding the value of some of Laing's early writing, his later work provided his critics with plenty of examples of arcane and pretentious prose, such as the following:

> if thoughts cannot be thought; and among the thoughts that cannot be thought is the thought that there are certain thoughts that cannot be thought, including the aforementioned thought, then he who has complied with this calculus of anti-thought will not be aware he is not aware that he is obeying a rule not to think that he is obeying a rule not to think about X.
>
> (Laing, 1972 in Sim, 1981: 585)

> At the point of nonbeing we are at the outer reaches of what language can state, but we can indicate by language why language cannot say what it cannot say. I cannot say what cannot be said, but sounds can make us listen to the silence.
>
> (Laing, 1967: 35)

While such elaborate word games are both clever and poetic, any valid observations they might contain are well hidden. Indeed they are more like the koans used as an aid to meditation by Zen Buddhists than the incisive insights of a radical psychiatrist. Thus they accentuate the image of Laing as some sort of guru and detract from the importance of his early work criticizing the cold detachment of medical psychiatry.

Thomas Szasz

At around the same time as Laing published *The Divided Self*, a psychiatrist in the USA named Thomas Szasz also published a book attacking medical psychiatry: *The Myth of Mental Illness* (Szasz, 1961). Ironically, although anti-psychiatry has often been caricatured as a left-wing attempt at politicizing mental health issues, the most detailed political analysis of mental health to date has been the right-wing libertarian perspective offered by Szasz. Like Laing, Szasz had begun to develop his ideas about mental health while doing compulsory military service as a psychiatrist during the 1950s, and had published some papers addressing these themes before the publication of his *magnum opus* (Kerr, 1997; Laing, 1994). However, whereas Laing's critique of psychiatry amounts to an impassioned plea for greater empathic understanding of mentally distressed persons, Szasz's argument is a direct attack on the legitimacy of both medical psychiatry and psychotherapy (Szasz, 1979a, 1979b). Moreover, Szasz has always expressed his intense irritation with those who have bracketed him together with Laing, Cooper *et al.*, who he accused of hypocrisy, naïvety and living off the society they condemn as 'schizophrenogenic' (Szasz, 1978, 1979b). His preferred description of himself is 'libertarian psychiatrist' and his principle concern is the injustice of psychiatric coercion (Szasz, 1994).

The central argument of *The Myth of Mental Illness* is that there is no substantive similarity between known physical illnesses and so-called mental illness such as schizophrenia and depression. The basis of this argument is that no organic cause can be positively identified for a person's communications about themselves, others and the world about them. Therefore, Szasz argues, the process of diagnosis in modern psychiatry may be likened to medieval examinations for signs of demonic possession. The present state examination which is at the centre of the diagnostic process is a search for phenomena which exist only in the imagination of psychiatrists themselves. Furthermore, as 'mental illness' is merely a social construction, the compulsory detention of distressed persons for 'treatment' is a total violation of their civil rights.

In later books he develops this analysis in a number of ways. He suggests that 'mental illness' is merely an excuse for wrongdoing that was invented to mitigate offenders' suffering at the hands of their accusers. He argues that the State has no business managing the private and moral problems of its citizens (Szasz, 1971). He also describes 'schizophrenics' as social nuisances with no respect for the rights of others and vilifies Laing for claiming to treat what he considers to be a non-existent ailment (i.e. schizophrenia) (Szasz, 1979b).

It is difficult to assess whether Szasz and Laing have had an equal impact on ideas about mental health, or whether one has been more significant than the other. Both have been marginalized by mainstream psychiatry, although inasmuch as he was a Professor of Psychiatry at the State University of New York from 1956 until 1990, Szasz did at least remain part of the psychiatric establishment (Kerr, 1997). Laing, on the other hand, was in independent practice from the mid-1960s onwards and never held a university teaching appointment. Szasz has certainly written more (over 20 books plus many journal articles compared to Laing's 15 books plus several journal articles). Moreover, all of Szasz's books are conventional academic books whereas Laing's oeuvre includes two books of poetry and one book which comprises transcripts of conversations with his own children. At the time of writing (1999), Szasz is still alive and still writing while Laing died in 1989. Whereas Laing's theoretical arguments were rooted in esoteric philosophies and expressed in poetic language, Szasz's arguments (although often intensely polemical and emotive) are usually based on thorough historical and theoretical research. Thus, Szasz's arguments often seem more convincing than those of either Laing or Cooper, both of whom could be lax in their approach to referencing their sources. However, *Encyclopaedia Britannica – CD 99* has an entry for Laing which credits him with developing a radical approach to the management of schizophrenia, but has no entry for Szasz.

Another key issue is that as Szasz was never really associated with the radical chic of the 1960s and 1970s, interest in him did not fade with the demise of the counter-culture. Indeed, his views about the politics of mental health are very close to the political agenda of the New Right, a political movement that was gaining popularity as the vaguely left-wing politics of the counter-culture was in decline (Green, 1987; Seldon, 1985). For example, Szasz's claim that psychiatry fosters a culture of dependency, and his attack on all forms of state-funded welfare provision are very much in tune with New Right thinking on the welfare state (Szasz, 1979b, 1994). Likewise, New Right criminologists have found that his critique of forensic psychiatry fits well with their views about social responsibility, crime and punishment (Tame, 1991).

While Szasz often attacked Laing and other members of the Philadelphia Association, Laing was apparently more tolerant of Szasz. For example, in interviews he gave during the 1980s Laing made the following comments about Szasz:

Now, in *Wisdom, Madness and Folly*, I can afford to adopt this sort of soft tone, in the book, because Szasz is in the world saying the sort of stuff that he is saying. I mean if there wasn't Thomas Szasz in the world I would have to invent him! I'd have to be that myself.

(Laing in Bigwood, 1990: 29)

I was very sad about [Szasz's criticism of me] because I thought that, although I could well imagine that Szasz had things that he would disagree with me about, that basically we were ... [on] something like the same side.

(Laing cited in Mullan, 1995: 202)

This contrasts sharply with Szasz's opinion of both Laing and Cooper:

Cooper has a heart that bleeds for victims, especially of his own imaginings. His compassion has become cancerous and has all but destroyed him. Laing, on the other hand, has a good sense for business – in particular, for selling his dramatized impersonations of himself. So far he has sold himself as student of schizophrenia, theoretician of anti-psychiatry, charismatic healer of madness, existential philosopher, New Leftist social critic, guru of LSD, Buddhist monk, and medical critic of the family ... Cooper is often wrong-headed, but is honest. Laing is often level-headed, but is he ever honest?

(Szasz, 1978: 73)

However, in spite of the differences between Szasz and the anti-psychiatrists, one concern they share is a distaste for psychiatric coercion and state control of mental health services. Furthermore, the anti-psychiatry of the Philadelphia Association and the libertarian psychiatry of Thomas Szasz both provide alternative frameworks for practice as well as critiques of mainstream medical psychiatry. For over 30 years the Philadelphia Association has provided a small network of therapeutic communities (usually referred to as 'houses') which provide an alternative to traditional hospital-based mental health care. Additionally, the Arbours Association has provided a similar network of houses run on similar principles since 1970. For many years, Thomas Szasz also practised what he preached, running a successful part-time psychotherapy practice based on the principles that all clients must refer themselves and pay for his services (Kerr, 1997).

While it is possible to identify a historical period during which several radical critiques (including those associated with Szasz and the Philadelphia Association) emerged alongside each other, the emergence of critiques of prevailing ideologies on mental health is not unique to this era. In the 1920s, Montagu Lomax's infamous attack on British psychiatry and British psychiatric hospitals resulted in reports in national newspapers, questions in Parliament and ultimately to the Royal Commission on Lunacy and Mental Disorder of 1924–1926 (Harding, 1990). It was also during the 1920s that the German psychoanalyst Wilhelm Reich became sceptical of the value of individual therapy. Accordingly, he spent many years working on the development of a holistic approach to mental health care which incorporated ideas about life force which he termed 'orgone energy' ('chi' or 'prana' as it is known in Chinese medicine and Indian yoga), psychoanalysis, sexuality and sociological analysis (Reich, 1975a). Moreover, although they never directly challenged mainstream thinking, Viktor Frankl, Bruno Bettelheim and Eugene Heimler developed new psychotherapeutic approaches because their own traumatic experiences in Nazi concentration camps had led them to question some of the assumptions of established psychiatric and psychoanalytical theories.

New wave critiques of therapy

New critiques of psychiatry and psychotherapy continue to emerge. For example, during the 1980s, a number of writers challenged some of the basic assumptions of psychiatry and psychotherapy. These include: the psychiatrist Peter Breggin who has attacked medical psychiatry; the former psychoanalyst Jeffrey Masson, who argues that psychotherapy is at best useless, and, at worst, abusive; the psychiatrist Marius Romme and the science journalist Sandra Escher whose ideas about voice-hearing have stimulated renewed debate about the nature of psychosis; and service users such as Louise Pembroke and Diane Harrison who have questioned psychiatric assumptions about the meaning of self-harm and how it should be managed.

Jeffrey Masson is probably the best known and most influential of these critics, not least because his work directly challenges the assumption that 'talking therapies' are a real alternative to medical psychiatry:

Therapists depend on a social network for referrals. So even if an individual therapist is completely opposed to somatic intervention

– drugs or electroshock, for example – working in a setting where these are used is often difficult to avoid, and the opposition then becomes internalized, i.e., silenced. This is another step along the road of corruption. And even those therapists who are not part of a hospital setting are nevertheless part of a larger [community of therapists] that will not take lightly any departure from professional solidarity.

(Masson, 1990: 296)

This is significant because, with the exception of David Cooper, the anti-psychiatrists believed in the value of some form of psychotherapy, and even Thomas Szasz is prepared to practise as a therapist as long as all his clients are voluntary and pay a fee. Thus, the implication of Masson's critique of therapy is that even mental health professionals who consider themselves to be radicals cannot afford to be complacent.

Masson is a former psychoanalyst and a former director of the Sigmund Freud archives who began to question the validity of psychotherapy when he realized that Freud had re-defined his clients' accounts of actual sexual abuse as 'wish-fulfilment fantasies' (Masson, 1984). To Masson this was only the first of many betrayals of the victims of human suffering by psychology, psychotherapy and psychiatry. In what is possibly his best known book, Masson reviews the life and work of several well-known therapists and shows how some of them have abused and exploited their clients, while others have been hopelessly ineffective (Masson, 1990). While he acknowledges that some people have been helped by some therapists, he attributes this to the personal qualities of individual therapists, rather than to the validity of psychotherapeutic theory and intervention (Masson, 1990).

Masson's critique of psychotherapy is complemented by Peter Breggin's critique of medical psychiatry. In his early work, Breggin sought to establish the malevolent nature of psychiatry by detailing how psychiatrists had willingly and actively participated in the extermination of mentally ill and learning disabled people in Nazi Germany (Breggin, 1973). While this is certainly true (Burleigh, 1994), it is unclear whether these psychiatrists acted in this way because they were first and foremost psychiatrists, or because they were first and foremost Nazis. If it were the latter, it is hardly fair to blame the psychiatric profession as a whole for their actions. Nevertheless, the fact that any psychiatrists could be persuaded to participate in such barbarity arguably compromises any claim that the practice of psychiatry is inherently altruistic and thus mirrors Masson's critique of psychotherapy and reinforces Szasz, Cooper and Laing's critiques of psychiatric coercion.

In his more recent work, Breggin (1993) has been less extreme, suggesting that the over-reliance of psychiatrists on drug treatments reflects the fact that psychiatry is more about social control than care of the mentally distressed. Although sceptical about the value of psychotherapy he warns would-be consumers of therapy that only they can judge whether their therapist is helping them. In these respects, his critique of psychiatry is not dissimilar to that of Thomas Szasz. However, whereas Szasz is enthusiastic about all forms of consumerism and the supposed virtues of free markets, Breggin implies that there is collaboration between the pharmaceutical industry and the psychiatric profession because of the mutual financial benefits which arise from this relationship (Breggin, 1993).

Marius Romme and Sandra Escher's perspective on the phenomenon of hearing voices (which psychiatry traditionally defines as auditory hallucinations) is not dissimilar to labelling theory. Labelling theory suggests that behaviour which is perceived as 'abnormal' provokes others to define the individual(s) exhibiting such behaviour as deviant. This reaction leads 'deviant' individuals to develop other 'deviant' behaviours in an effort to cope with this stigmatization, so that the label of 'deviant' effectively becomes a self-fulfilling prophecy. A detailed analysis of how labelling theory may explain 'mental illness' was provided in the 1960s by the American sociologist Thomas Scheff (1966) and was also a submerged theme in the work of David Cooper and R. D. Laing.

Romme and Escher argue that people who hear voices are stigmatized in this way and that any distress that their voices might cause them is amplified when others attempt to define the meaning of the voices for them or claim that their voices are meaningless (Romme and Escher, 1993). One of the most important aspects of Romme and Escher's work has been their involvement with a Dutch television programme about voice-hearing in the mid-1980s. This resulted in 700 persons responding to an appeal to contact them. Of these, 450 reported hearing voices, 150 of whom had developed strategies for coping with their voices and/or had never been in contact with psychiatric services. The importance of these findings is that they led Romme and Escher to question the assumption of many psychiatrists that hearing multiple voices or hearing voices commenting on one's own thoughts and actions are diagnostic of 'schizophrenia' (Rose, 1992). Later research by Romme and Escher has led them to conclude that voices usually represent unresolved problems or traumas, and the aim of therapy should be to stimulate curiosity about the content of a person's voices so that resolution may be achieved (Romme and Escher, 1996). Thus Romme and Escher have stimulated investigation of the value of cognitive-behavioural interventions in managing so-called psychotic disorders (e.g. Haddock and Slade, 1996) and have inspired the national self-help and advocacy organization, the Hearing Voices Network, which was formed in 1990 (Baker, 1993; Grierson, 1991).

However, although the work of Romme and Escher should not be underestimated, they are not the first researchers to make such a discovery, and neither are cognitive therapists the first to develop psychological methods of managing psychotic experiences (Schatzman, *circa* 1980). The significance of Romme and Escher's work is that it coincided with the rise of a mental health service users' movement which, after many years of struggle, was at last being taken seriously by mental health professionals and had grown significantly since the mid-1980s (Campbell, 1991; 'Seeger', 1996). Thus, the emergence of the Hearing Voices Network is representative of a wider pattern of mental health service users directly challenging psychiatric ideology by publicizing recent qualitative and quantitative research findings. Another example of this is the formation of a National Self-Harm Network.

Self-harm is a behaviour which has often been misunderstood, misinterpreted and treated unsympathetically (even brutally) by members of the psychiatric profession (Harrison, 1995; Pembroke, 1994). However, until the publication of Louise Pembroke's (1994) edited collection of accounts by self-harmers (*Self-Harm: Perspectives from Personal Experience*), user-centred accounts of self-harm were rare. Since the publication of this excellent ground-breaking book, other books addressing similar themes have followed including Diane Harrison's (1995) detailed exploration of women and self-harm in society, *Vicious Circles*, while a National Self-Harm Network has also been established. Louise Pembroke was one of the prime movers in establishing this network which campaigns for greater professional understanding of self-harm (for example, Pembroke *et al.*, 1996).

Fred Newman and the East Side Institute for Short Term Psychotherapy

One other approach to mental health which should also be mentioned here is the so-called 'Social Therapy' practised by Fred Newman, Lois

Holzman and their associates at the East Side Institute for Short Term Psychotherapy. (It should be noted that when Newman and Holzman use the term 'Social Therapy' they are not referring to the approach to social psychiatry adopted by liberal psychiatrists such as David Clark, but to a specific form of group therapy based on ideas borrowed from Wittgenstein, Marx and Vygotsky.) Newman has never been a mental health professional or mental health service user. He is a self-styled political activist and a former philosophy lecturer. In this sense, he stands apart from the others whose work is discussed in this chapter. However, inasmuch as he is the 'inventor' of Social Therapy he is a therapist, while his close associate Holzman is a qualified developmental psychologist. Although Newman claims that his 'Social Therapy' is a Marxist therapy, there are several reasons for discussing it in this chapter rather than elsewhere. First, Newman claims that Social Therapy is an 'anti-therapy', and for this reason alone it should be considered alongside 'anti-psychiatry' (Newman, 1991). Second, inasmuch as it arises from a critique of medical psychiatry and clinical psychology and views mental distress as a socio-political rather than an individual problem, it shares common ground with 'anti-psychiatry', particularly the work of David Cooper (Newman, 1991; Parker, 1995). Third, many Far Left organizations in the USA are suspicious of the East Side Institute for Short Term Psychotherapy (and its sister organizations, the Castillo Center and the New Alliance Party) and are sceptical of Newman's claim to be a *bona fide* Marxist (Parker, 1995). In this sense, it may be more appropriate to think of Newman and his colleagues as radical therapists rather than political activists.

Newman claims that Social Therapy is radically different from any other form of group therapy and, at first sight this claim does not seem unreasonable. After all, Newman and his colleagues have inspired others to open Social Therapy centres in at least seven other North American cities and have attracted the interest of self-styled radical psychologists in Europe (Parker, 1995). Furthermore, Newman and Holzman's (1993a) arguments against psychiatry and other forms of psychotherapy are persuasive. They argue that it is impossible to understand another person's emotions; that psychotherapy merely teaches a person a new vocabulary to describe their emotional experience better but does not help them resolve psychological and emotional problems; and that mental health professionals should concentrate on enabling people to create their own environments for learning and creativity. On the other hand, beneath the persuasive philosophical and theoretical arguments, the actual practice of Social Therapy seems to consist of little more than therapists and service users working together to raise funds to ensure the survival of the East Side Institute for Short Term Psychotherapy (Newman and Holzman, 1993b; Parker, 1995). This seems very similar to the activity of many communities which seek to establish alternative lifestyles (Bunker *et al.*, 1997) and is not dissimilar to the activities of many non-conformist Christian churches.

Moreover, traditional therapeutic communities which are located within statutory services and some charitable organizations are environments which foster creativity and learning without putting residents under pressure to raise funds to ensure the continued existence of those communities (see Kennard, 1998; Kennard and Roberts, 1983). Thus, while the members of the East Side Institute for Short Term Psychotherapy offer a new *theoretical* critique of medical psychiatry and mainstream psychology, their claim to have developed a radically new approach to group therapy is open to question. Logically, becoming an active member of any therapeutic community or self-supporting community might be expected to achieve the same therapeutic outcomes. Indeed, an authentic 'anti-therapy' or 'post-therapeutics' – particularly a Marxist one – would not advocate the creation of a community bound together only by a shared understanding of mental health and mental distress. Instead, it would be more orientated to straightforward community development initiatives.

Related critiques

Finally, the work of some anti-racist psychiatrists and some feminist critics of psychiatry and therapy overlaps with aspects of these other critical perspectives on mental health. For example, the anti-racist psychiatrist S. P. (Sashi) Sashidharan (1994) has invoked the work of Vygotsky, as well as the work of Fanon, in his analysis of how the coercive powers of psychiatry are used disproportionately against black people. In this sense, his analysis of medical psychiatry has things in common with Newman and Holzman's Social Therapy and the work of Laing, Cooper and Szasz.

An example of a feminist critique which overlaps with other critical perspectives is the lesbian-feminist critique of psychology offered by Kitzinger and Perkins (1993). This incorporates a critique of the way in which the vocabulary of psychotherapy has become part of everyday conversation, and the argument that the institutionalization of therapy has led to the redefinition of basic human qualities such as warmth, genuineness and empathy as specialist therapeutic skills. These observations echo Newman's assertion that much psychotherapy consists of elaborate word-games which do not help people resolve their personal crises, and Masson's claim that mentally distressed people need trustworthy confidantes, not self-styled professionals who make spurious claims to expertise in the management of other people's distress.

While there are overlaps between the various critical perspectives on mental health which are reviewed in this chapter (as well as between these and anti-racist and feminist perspectives), many of these are coincidental. Indeed, the only critical perspectives which are explicitly connected with each other are those of Laing, Cooper, other members of the Philadelphia Association and members of the Arbours Association. Even then, there are some major differences between the perspectives of Laing and Cooper, while there are also significant differences between the therapeutic philosophies which inform the work of the Philadelphia and Arbours Associations in the 1990s and the therapeutic philosophies which informed their work in the 1960s and 1970s.

Notwithstanding the changes that have taken place in the Philadelphia and Arbours Associations, some of their members are former colleagues of Laing and Cooper. The fact that they have chosen to work outside mainstream mental health services suggests that while anti-psychiatry made relatively little impact on mainstream ideologies of mental heath, it should be regarded as something more than a passing fad. Likewise, the close relationship of Szasz's philosophy of mental health to the politics of the New Right suggests that his work is also of continuing relevance. Since 1979, the politics of the New Right led to far-reaching change throughout British society including changes in social and political attitudes towards 'deviance' and publicly funded health and welfare services. Indeed, it may not be a coincidence that the gradual acceptance of the legitimacy of a mental health service users' movement coincided with the imposition of market principles and consumerist principles on the health and welfare services. Furthermore, it is not unusual for representatives of the mental health service users' movement to invoke Szasz's work in support of their critique of psychiatric coercion.

At first sight the work of David Cooper appears to be very dated. In a post-HIV world where safe sex is the norm, his apologias for sexual libertarianism seem quaint examples of 1960s optimism. In a society which has been changed so radically by eighteen continuous years of right-wing governments that Tony Blair's New Labour government is not left-wing but 'right of centre', his appeals to revolutionary Marxism also seem like relics of a faintly remembered past. On the other hand, the existence of the East Side Institute of Short Term Psychotherapy and Fred Newman's claim that the therapy practised there is a Marxist therapy, suggests that some of Cooper's ideas may be of continuing relevance.

Admittedly, such critical perspectives have always been marginalized by the mainstream mental health professions. However, there are still numerically small coalitions of mental health professionals and mental health service users whose members take these perspectives seriously. For example, the newsletter of the radical psychology group, Psychology Politics Resistance (aka PPR – founded in 1994), and the low circulation magazine for democratic psychiatry, *Asylum* (founded in 1986), often carry articles which refer to these perspectives. Similarly, many young students who are introduced to the ideas of Laing and Szasz today are interested in these perspectives and are willing to explore their relevance to the contemporary situation. On the other hand, it would be extremely unusual to find a mental health professional who claimed to be applying a Laingian approach in his/her daily work, even though many who entered the mental health professions during the 1960s and 1970s may have been influenced by anti-psychiatry to some extent. Furthermore, any attempt to understand the meaning of psychotic experiences owes something to the work of the anti-psychiatrists, while the debate about care and control was first articulated by both Szasz and the anti-psychiatrists in their critiques of psychiatric coercion.

A more detailed analysis of the inter-relationship between various critical perspectives on mental health, and their continuing relevance at the turn of the twentieth and twenty-first century is undertaken in Chapter 7. The following chapter focuses on the impact of anti-racism and feminism on theories of mental health and distress and the practice of mental health care. Although there was not an explicit anti-racist or feminist dimension to anti-psychiatry, the emergence of new feminist and anti-racist perspectives on mental health and mental distress from the mid-1970s onwards reflects the social and political significance of the counter-culture of which anti-psychiatry was a part. This was essentially about challenging a world order based on capitalist accumulation, patriarchal rule, neo-colonialism and narrow-mindedness. Thus discourses of feminism and anti-racism were a product of the counter-culture, while anti-psychiatry (which was itself linked to the counter-culture) encouraged the critical examination of discourses of mental health and mental distress. Thus, there is a connection between anti-psychiatry and later feminist and anti-racist perspectives on mental health, mental distress and mental health care.

5 Gender and race critiques of psychiatry

It was primarily the critical perspectives which emerged in the 1960s and 1970s that exposed mental health and mental illness as highly controversial and heavily contested categories. These perspectives located 'madness' in socio-politics; refuted the concept of madness as 'illness'; and questioned the power of psychiatrists to act as arbiters of 'normality' and 'abnormality'. Once it was established that what constitutes 'madness' is fluctuating and ambiguous, then it became possible to theorize how mental disorder is related to social divisions based on class, race, ethnicity, gender, sexuality and age. Whereas differences in patterns of mental health and illness had traditionally been attributed to the inherently flawed 'nature' or vulnerability of certain individuals or groups, attention turned to the significance of oppressive social relations and the social construction of health and illness.

This chapter explores these perspectives in relation to the differential experiences of women and black and minority ethnic groups in the mental health system. There is a conscious effort to emphasize the complexity and interconnectedness of processes of discrimination and oppression in people's lives, recognizing that while reality is experienced at the level of the individual, it is important to construct theories and policies which enable action at the social and structural levels. Such an approach is in keeping with the current demand for the mental health system and professionals within it to become more sensitive to the dynamics of discrimination and oppression and the expressed needs of people in mental distress.

Gender and mental distress

Facts and figures

For the past twenty-five years it has been feminist writers from a wide range of backgrounds who have primarily been responsible for opening up the terrain of gender and madness to wider debate (Chesler, 1972; Ehrenreich and English, 1979; Miles, 1988; Orbach, 1979, 1993; Penfold and Walker, 1984; Russell, 1995; Showalter, 1987; Ussher, 1991). Most have taken as their starting point the over-representation of women as patients in the mental health system. From here they are variously concerned to first, explain how they got there and second, document their oppressive treatment within the system. However, this starting point is itself problematic. While many subscribe to the view that 'madness' is a distinctively female malady, citing statistical data in support of this conclusion (Briscoe, 1982; Gove, 1979; Showalter, 1987) Joan Busfield argues that when the epidemiological data is disaggregated:

> the picture is far more complex, and the actual female predomi-nance is far from monolithic ... It is not so much that mental disorder overall is a female malady, but that some mental disor-ders appear to be more distinctively female, whilst others have a more masculine face, and yet others are more or less gender-neutral.
>
> (1996: 14)

Measures of mental disorder are primarily constructed from patient statistics and community surveys. Such data consistently shows that anorexia nervosa, anxiety and depression are predominantly female diagnoses. Studies indicate that more than 90 per cent of cases of anorexia occur in women (American Psychiatric Association, 1994), while community surveys of anxiety and depression generally indicate a 2:1 ratio (Goldberg and Huxley, 1980; Weissman and Klerman, 1977). Yet there are a range of disorders where gender differences are less clear cut, namely schizophrenia, mania and psychotic depression. Explanations for these gendered patterns are, of course, contentious. Initially there are issues to do with the limitations of the methodologies used to measure mental disorder. Indeed there is a wealth of literature concerning the problems of both defining and measuring mental ill health (see, for example, Dohrenwend and Dohrenwend, 1969; Laing, 1959; Payne, 1991). Busfield (1996) argues first, that the variability in definitions and measures of disorder between studies makes comparability between them poor. It appears that the definition of mental illness will depend on which measure is being used and by whom. Second, the vagaries of institutional practices and the exclusion of untreated cases makes patient statistics unreliable. Third, screening devices are often gender-biased, demonstrating selectivity in sets of disorders and constructions of selected disorders. Finally, self-reports reflect cultural biases in terms of the acceptability of certain expressions of mental distress.

Due to these limitations, Busfield concludes that there can be no universal generalization that mental disorder is more common in women than men. The whole idea of establishing true rates of prevalence or incidence is, she argues, something of a chimera. Epidemiological findings must be treated as construct-specific – that is, if the boundaries of mental disorder are changed, then the gender balance is also likely to change. Moreover, epidemiological data are social products which 'tell us more about psychiatric practices and the mental health system than they do about gender differences in mental health problems' (Busfield, 1996: 9). This suggests that the problems go much deeper than statistical inaccuracies. Feminist analyses have highlighted the need to examine how the construction of disease categories themselves, biases in psychiatric assessment, and the socialization of gendered psychologies, all contribute to an understanding of gender and mental health. There are a number of different positions in feminist theorizing on women's madness, ranging from madness as a female issue to madness as a feminist issue.

Just labelling women crazy?

Following social constructionist perspectives is the suggestion that madness is not an illness but a label attached to women who step outside of the boundaries of acceptable femininity. In this it is argued that notions of correct feminine behaviour have helped to shape expectations and understandings of women's mental distress for those who use mental health services and for those who provide such services. As with other critiques opposed to psychiatry, such analyses point to the significance of power structures in defining madness. However, for feminist writers these power structures are clearly patriarchal and this helps to explain why women are over-represented as 'mad'. Phyllis Chesler in her influential study *Women and Madness* argues that gender is embedded in the very construction of concepts of madness and mental illness:

What we consider 'madness', whether it appears in women or in men, is either the acting out of the devalued female role or the total or partial rejection of one's sex-role stereotype.

(1972: 56)

Therefore, it is suggested that the simple act of departing from the roles expected of men and women in a patriarchal society can lead to definitions of disorder. However for women there is a double bind. In patriarchal society masculinity is privileged and femininity devalued. Therefore women who both conform to or depart from their sex-role stereotype are liable to attract diagnoses of mental disorder. Thus women fall prey to the paradox that constructs them as mad or pathological if they accept or reject prevailing norms of femininity (Penfold and Walker, 1984; Ussher, 1991).

Madness and asylums generally function as mirror images of the female experience, and penalties for being 'female', as well as for desiring or daring not to be.

(Chesler, 1972: 16)

In support of this assertion, Chesler cites the well-known study by Broverman *et al.* (1970) which examined clinicians' conceptions of mental health. This study not only demonstrated the operation of gender-based stereotypes in conceptions of mental health and illness, but also that the assessment of what constitutes a mentally healthy adult (sex unspecified) corresponds most closely with the prevailing masculine stereotype. Psychological ill health was consistently associated with the feminine stereotype. A number of other studies have confirmed that mental health professionals are more likely to equate feminine characteristics with mental ill health (Corob, 1987; Penfold and Walker, 1984; Sheppard, 1991; Weissman and Klerman, 1977). In this sense the social construction of women as essentially mad is considered to be one more manifestation of the way in which women are controlled within patriarchy. The labelling process is seen as functioning to maintain women's position as outsiders; dismiss women's anger as illness; and explain women's unhappiness as some internal flaw. This obscures any attempt to question the social structures of patriarchy. Moreover, this process has been seen to operate over time, the labels changing according to prevailing discourses. Thus, for example, Showalter (1987) argues that Victorian discourses around femininity produced constructions of women's deviancy which were labelled as hysteria or neurasthenia, while in the twentieth century these have been replaced by labels such as anxiety, depression and anorexia.

Biology as destiny

It is the connection of women's madness with biology that is identified by many feminist writers as the most powerful discourse bearing down on women (Ehrenreich and English, 1979; Showalter, 1987). As the discourse of madness as illness began to predominate during the nineteenth century, justifications for women's exclusion took on a distinctly medical character. Buttressed by scientific rhetoric, madness was associated with femininity and with the female body. In particular there was an obsession with the perceived dangerousness of women's unbridled sexuality. Foucault (1967: 104) notes how 'the female body was analyzed – qualified and disqualified – as being thoroughly saturated with sexuality; whereby it was integrated into the sphere of medical practices, by reason of a pathology intrinsic to it'. Masturbation, illegitimate pregnancy, homosexuality, frigidity, promiscuity and nymphomania were embraced within an illness framework, seen as symptoms or forms of insanity. While men were also diagnosed with 'disorders' arising from their supposed 'unnatural sexuality' (such as the diagnosis of 'masturbatory insanity'), and thereby equally liable to incarceration in asylums, it was women who experienced some of the most severe 'treatments' such as clitoridectomy.

Given the bias towards biologism in psychiatry at this time and the view that heredity was the primary source of insanity, it is hardly surprising that women's reproductive systems became the focus of the medical men. Ordinary functions of the female life cycle such as menstruation, pregnancy and the menopause were pathologized and psychiatrized. Skultans cites a typical physician's ideas on the subject of the menopause:

> The critical period, as it is called, when menstruation ceases, is certainly a period favourable to the development of mental aberration.
>
> (1975: 224)

As Jane Ussher (1991: 74/75) notes 'madness was almost inevitable, given the female constitution' and it was hysteria which 'became the accepted diagnosis of all aspects of female madness, as well as a whole cornucopia of other female maladies'.

Biological explanations of women's madness have continued to dominate mental health theory and practice throughout the twentieth century. As in the nineteenth century, the emphasis is on reproductive biology, in particular women's genetic and hormonal tendency to mental disorder (for example, pre-menstrual tension (PMT) or syndrome (PMS); post-natal depression and menopausal syndrome). However, although the science has become more sophisticated, the evidence of any direct links between reproductive biology and specific mental disorders (in either men or women) is poor. Indeed, while findings are largely inconsistent with hypotheses derived from the biological approach to women's madness (Kaufert *et al.*, 1992; McFarlane and Williams, 1994; McKinlay *et al.*, 1987; Nicolson, 1992; Walker, 1995), nevertheless research and practice grounded in this perspective continues unabated. In this sense, feminist writers suggest it is likely that the over-emphasis on biologically based theories of gender differences in mental health reflects sexist assumptions and ideologies more than scientific fact (Birke, 1986; Caplan *et al.*, 1992; Edwards, 1988; Laws, 1985; Nicolson, 1986, 1990, 1991; O'Sullivan, 1982; Ussher, 1989, 1992).

This is not to suggest that biology is insignificant, but that the attribution of meaning to biological and physical processes reflects 'culturally specific assumptions' (Parker *et al.*, 1995: 15). For example, with regards to PMS, there is a marked lack of consensus about its defining characteristics. Although 'the material processes associated with the menstrual cycle are a universal physical experience for the vast majority of women of reproductive age' (Swann, 1997: 176), Western attitudes to it have been shaped primarily within the context of medical knowledge and technologies. In particular, the menstrual cycle has increasingly been identified as a psycho-medical 'problem', to the extent that PMS is included in the latest edition of the Diagnostic and Statistical Manual of the American Psychiatric Association (APA, 1994) as 'Late Luteal Phase Dysphoric Disorder'. Why should there be a problem in accepting the notion that there may be cyclical changes in women's (or indeed men's) moods, levels of aggression or sexual desire? More significantly, why are particular manifestations of such changes constructed negatively? Swann contends that PMS research needs to move away from the limitations of the biological model, towards an account that allows for the significance of culture, gender and power, and their relationship to lived experience. Power and knowledge structure the way human beings understand 'health' and 'illness' and the relationship between physical and mental distress (Zola, 1972). Beliefs and expectations may produce experiences of our bodily states which may fluctuate, as those beliefs and expectations themselves change. Therefore experiences of mental distress cannot simply be reduced to biology.

Made mad through patriarchy?

Another distinctive line in feminist theorizing on gender and mental distress acknowledges the existence of women's madness but explains it as a function of living in an oppressive patriarchal society. Such approaches emphasize the significance of the social circumstances of women's everyday lives, including gendered sources of stress and their impact on women (Stoppard, 1997: 10). The particular stresses women are exposed to – economic dependence; familial caring responsibilities; social isolation; physical and sexual abuse; the politics of appearance – have all been identified as significant factors making them vulnerable to mental distress (see, for example, Brown and Harris, 1978; Burnam *et al.*, 1988; Coward, 1984; Dobash and Dobash, 1979; Finch and Groves, 1983; Finch and Mason, 1992; Graham, 1993; Jehu, 1990; Koss, 1990; McFarland, 1991; MacLeod, 1981; Oakley, 1976; Orbach, 1979, 1993; Payne, 1991; Sharpe, 1984; Sluka, 1989; Surrey *et al.*, 1990; Wolf, 1990).

It is suggested that women are not only socially disadvantaged by the roles they are expected to perform but also psychologically disadvantaged by the socialization processes that prepare them for these roles. Many feminists, having rejected biologically deterministic arguments of the origins of women's mental distress, have looked to psychological theories to explain the development of gendered psychologies. Although critical of the sexist nature of Freud's ideas on women and sexuality, feminist theorizing on male and female psychology has primarily evolved within a psychodynamic framework. Indeed until the 1970s, most feminists viewed Freud with hostility. They challenged the content and practice of psychoanalysis arguing that it was inherently sexist because of its emphasis on biology over social relations (Friedan, 1963) and the fact that it took masculine characteristics as a psychoanalytic norm (de Beauvoir, 1972). But while many feminists condemned Freud himself, few made the distinction between the man and the subsequent use of his ideas.

By 1974 Juliet Mitchell, a Marxist feminist, became a major force in convincing feminists of the relevance and value of psychoanalysis for feminism. She argued that although psychoanalytic *practice* could be seen as a patriarchal institution, serving the prevailing values of patriarchal culture, psychoanalytic *theory* could nevertheless provide an explanation for patriarchal power relations that is profoundly threatening to those relations (Rowley and Grosz, 1992). Strongly influenced by the work of the French anthropologist Levi-Strauss and the French psychoanalyst Jacques Lacan, Mitchell argued that feminists had been placing Freud's ideas in a false context. This, she suggested, had led them to neglect or dismiss the valuable insights his work offers into the complex psychological processes by which gender identity is shaped through patriarchy from earliest childhood:

> Where Marxist theory explains the historical and economic situation, psychoanalysis, in conjunction with the notions of ideology already gained by dialectical materialism, is the way into understanding ideology and sexuality.

> (Mitchell, 1974: xxii)

By contrast, other feminists (such as Chodorow, 1978; Dinnerstein, 1976; Eichenbaum and Orbach, 1982; Orbach, 1979; Rich, 1976) have drawn upon the object-relations school of psychoanalytic theory characterized by the work of Melanie Klein and Donald Winnicott. These feminists contend that women's oppression and women's mental distress can be understood through an examination of patterns of childbearing and rearing. Dorothy Dinnerstein (1976: 111) argues, 'so long as the first parent is a woman, then, woman will be inevitably pressed into the dual role of indispensable quasi-human supporter and deadly quasi-human enemy of the self'. She points to the enduring nature of men's and women's fears and fantasies about their mothers. Similarly, Nancy Chodorow (1978: 9) has examined the effects of mothering on the identity and psychological make-up of women and men suggesting that 'women's mothering is a central and defining feature of the social organization of gender and is implicated in the construction and organization of male dominance itself'. Chodorow argues that psychoanalysis may be able to explain how mothering is reproduced from generation to generation without any observable coercion. Her use of psychoanalysis is more overtly clinical than Mitchell's, offering a set of empirical insights into men's and women's lives, experiences and behaviours that may contribute to progressive social and political changes. In particular, the advocacy of 'collective child-rearing' is seen as having 'far-reaching implications for every aspect of women's experience, madness included' (Ussher, 1991: 200). Object-relations theory has also influenced the approach to mental health practice developed by Louise Eichenbaum and Susie Orbach

(1982, 1984) at the Women's Therapy Centres founded in London and New York.

Diversity and difference

Increasingly within feminist analyses it has been recognized that it is not good enough to simply focus on the universal category of 'woman', as this does not reflect the diversity of experience within that category. As Rieker and Jankowski state:

> As a routine aspect of daily life sexism intersects with racial and cultural differences to shape women's experience, identity, and psychological well-being.
>
> (1995: 27)

Racism, poverty and isolation shape the lives, opportunities and experiences of black and ethnic minority women who use mental health services. In the mainstream literature and practice the specific needs of these women are invisible (Commission for Racial Equality, 1992) and are only recognized and catered for in marginal contexts where there is a commitment to the provision of racially sensitive mental health services (Ismail, 1996; Mills, 1996). Racism also impacts on the lives of black and ethnic minority women who provide mental health services (Fenton and Sadiq, 1991).

Clearly women in mental distress live their lives within a whole range of determining contexts. To this end it is encouraging to see that there has been a growth in research, writing and practice which reflects the complexities of experiences of mental distress, for example for girls (Subotsky, 1996), older women (Livingston and Blanchard, 1996), black women (Ismail, 1996; Mills, 1996), lesbian women (Kitzinger and Perkins, 1993; O'Connor and Ryan, 1993; Perkins, 1996) and homeless women (Cook and Marshall, 1996). Nevertheless, it is disappointing that there continues to be a distinct lack of such material relating to the experiences of gay men and transsexuals (exceptions include Davies and Neal, 1996; Griggs, 1998; MacFarlane, 1998).

Women's experiences in the mental health system

Taken together, these various perspectives support the assertion that the mental health system is imbued with sexist ideology and therefore discriminates against women in mental distress. It is argued that, although largely well intentioned, mental health professionals locate problems within women and ignore or deny the socio-political factors that are the context, and frequently the source, of their distress. Many have double standards of mental health which have negative consequences for women (Chesler, 1972; Ehrenreich and English, 1974, 1976, 1979; Roberts, 1985). Chesler states:

> Clinicians, most of whom are men, all too often treat their patients, most of whom are women, as 'wives' and 'daughters', rather than as people: treat them as if female misery, by biological definition, exists outside the realm of what is considered human or adult.
>
> (1972: xxi)

The dominance of medical discourse in women's lives as a whole has been mirrored in the response to women's mental health. The connection of women's madness with biology has legitimated 'treatments' from clitoridectomy, sterilization, hysterectomy, through to lobotomy, insulin therapy, electro-convulsive therapy (ECT) and psychotropic medication. Women are twice as likely to be prescribed psychotropic medication (Cooperstock, 1981; Ettore and Riska, 1993; Penfold and Walker, 1984), and are more likely to receive ECT (Breggin, 1979; Buchan *et al.*, 1992; Knibbs, 1994). Ussher (1991) argues that many of these treatments, particularly the brain-disabling effects of ECT and lobotomy, have been used to literally reduce women to a child-like dependent state. Showalter (1987) claims that some psychiatric textbooks in the 1970s recommended lobotomy to enable a woman cope with her marriage.

Barrett and Roberts (1978: 42) showed how GPs tended to see middle-aged women in terms of their families and men in terms of their occupations. They found GPs extensively 'smoothed away surface anxieties' and adjusted women to a domestic life. Thousands of women have had relatively low levels of emotional distress transformed into serious drug dependency problems through the cavalier prescribing of minor tranquillizers by GPs misinformed by drug companies (Lacey and Woodward, 1985). While the recommendation from the Committee on the Safety of Medicines indicated that minor tranquillizers should be taken for no more than four weeks, some of these women had been prescribed them for ten or twenty years. In a study of referrals by GPs for compulsory mental health admissions, Sheppard (1991) found that GPs discriminated against women, referring considerably more women than men and for less severe mental disorders. This clearly raises important issues regarding the civil liberties of female patients.

Although at one level psychotherapy potentially represents a more caring and less invasive form of treatment it is not gender-neutral. As Juliet Mitchell states:

> There seems overwhelming justification for the charge that the many psychotherapeutic practices, including those that by the formal definition are within psychoanalysis, have done much to re-adapt discontented women to a conservative feminine status quo, to an inferiorized psychology and to a contentment with serving and servicing men and children.
>
> (1974: 299)

Feminist writers have been critical of the way in which women's oppression is transformed into illness in the therapeutic process (Ussher, 1991) and women are encouraged to look inwardly for the source of their distress rather than to the wider social structure. Mary Daly (1979) is uncompromising in her condemnation of therapy as 'mind rape'. Furthermore, research has documented women's experiences of sexual oppression by male therapists ranging from patronizing comments to sexual harassment, assault and rape (Chesler, 1972; Davidson, 1984; Masson, 1990; MIND, 1993; Rutter, 1995).

Feminist therapy

As a response to the inadequacies of mainstream psychological and psychiatric practice some feminists have sought to develop woman-centred, non-sexist therapies (Eichenbaum and Orbach, 1982, 1984; Ernst and Goodison, 1981; Holland, 1992; Hunter and Kelso, 1985; Watson and Williams, 1992). There is no one specific technique that characterizes these approaches, indeed they draw on a number of frameworks – psychoanalytic, behavioural, cognitive and humanistic – and function with individuals or groups. However, they share the same starting point – an acknowledgement of women's genuine distress which is not attributed to some inherent weakness or illness, but is seen as a response to their experiences of powerlessness. Consequently, there is a commitment to establishing an egalitarian therapeutic relationship which encourages empowerment and the restoration of women's self-esteem. As well as aiming for client-defined personal change there is a commitment to social and political action (Watson and Williams, 1992).

Some have questioned whether any therapy, including feminist therapy, is desirable (Masson, 1990). Jane Ussher (1991) argues that the gap between theory and practice in feminist therapy is wide and potentially hazardous. Since it draws on many of the same theoretical frameworks as traditional therapy it is hard to see how feminist therapy can avoid many of the same criticisms. It is still essentially a white, middle-class treatment that alienates black and working-class women. Moreover, how egalitarian can a therapeutic relationship really be when professional structures militate against genuine equality? Clearly it is not possible to simply wish power relationships away. Nevertheless, Chesler (1990) argues that women can and do benefit from feminist therapy – particularly when in crisis – and many are offered immediate sanctuary, practical and emotional support, and advocacy services every day in Women's Aid Centres, Rape Crisis Centres etc. throughout the country.

Limitations of the feminist perspectives

As with social constructionist approaches in general, some of the feminist positions have been criticized for being overly simplistic and one-dimensional. Women's distress is more than just a label – it is a real experience. To reduce this distress to mere social construction is not good enough. Some feminist accounts have not gone much beyond re-labelling madness as deviance. While there is real value in interpretative paradigms insofar as they allow us to make sense of the context of human behaviour from the point of view of the individual, there are limitations to their usefulness. For example, there is a danger in seeing women's 'symptoms' of mental distress as merely a form of protest in a patriarchal society. To suggest that this is emancipatory is highly questionable. Moreover, it infers that the individual woman consciously chose to express her protest in this way rather than some other. Certainly to account for all psychiatric diagnoses in such terms seems ludicrous. Ingleby (1981) suggests that we are still left with the 'so what?' problem as such frameworks are unable to account for 'residual mental disorder'. To a certain extent psychoanalytic approaches within feminism appear to remedy this problem of individual agency insofar as they recognize unconscious motives. However, as Ingleby (1981: 65) states, the excessive flexibility of such approaches makes them 'capable of encompassing everything and therefore explaining nothing'.

Equally problematic is the concept of an all-pervasive patriarchy within which women's mental health is constructed by psychiatrists acting as complicit agents of their social control. This presents an extremely pessimistic vision for women and completely denies the possibility of individual agency. In one sense it could be argued that all some feminist accounts have done is shift the locus of responsibility for women's madness from a deterministic 'nature' to a deterministic 'patriarchy'. Hilary Allen (1986) argues that in this respect some feminist analyses are polemical and empirically difficult to substantiate. She says that this is not to deny that psychiatry can be sexist, normative and guilty of abusing women, but that it is not legitimate or helpful to claim that it is intrinsically so. Further criticism levelled at feminist perspectives is that they only focus on women. While it is true that feminist approaches have had a crucial part to play in making women's experiences visible, there is a need to move beyond this to a fuller understanding of men's and women's experiences of mental distress, including the experiences of those who choose other expressions of sexuality. All are affected by deficiencies in the mental health system.

Despite the limitations of some feminist perspectives, the fact remains that complex processes of sex bias and sex-role stereotyping continue to detract from the quality of mental health services to *both* sexes. There is enough evidence to support the observation that the large volume of critical research about women, men and mental health has not been incorporated into mental health training so that mental health workers' knowledge in this area is inadequate. Busfield (1996) argues that possibilities for action only begin to emerge when we recognize the way in which gender permeates categories of mental disorder. The most obvious course of action is to shift mental health practice away from its strongly individualizing mould in which the individual is pathologized, to a frame of reference which accepts and recognizes the importance of social and material circumstances in shaping men's and women's lives and their mental health. The inadequacies can be remedied by organizations developing services for users which are based on thorough assessments of the users' needs and from a 'new' understanding of men's and women's behaviour. In order to do this properly, service providers need to listen to users, train staff to be sensitive to gender differences and operate equal opportunities policies. Women's groups, service users and mental health workers who advocate gender-sensitive services are beginning to make an impact on how diagnosis and treatment is being delivered (Abel *et al.*, 1996) but more dialogue is needed.

Johnson and Buszewicz (1996) summarize a number of key issues which need to be addressed in the development of gender sensitive mental health services:

- Services must be equally accessible to all groups of men and women. They should be able to feel safe and comfortable in the setting where the service is delivered.
- Women's access to power must be enhanced in order to improve their self-esteem.
- A full range of services must be available to men and women, not just drug treatments.
- There is a need to plan with diversity of experiences in mind, recognizing the variety of contexts in which people live their lives.
- Services must be developed in consultation with users, carers and the voluntary sector organizations.
- There needs to be a commitment to investing in staff – including training and development and the provision of good working conditions to avoid 'burnout'.

Race, ethnicity and mental distress

As with feminist critiques, the starting point for critiques of the mental health system based on analyses of race and ethnicity is often a concern with the epidemiology of madness. However, the statistical data on race, ethnicity and mental health is even more problematic than for gender. The Department of Health has not systematically collected statistics indicating the racial or ethnic background of psychiatric patients. Any ethnic monitoring that does take place in the statutory services tends to be patchy and sporadic. Independent research studies have attempted to fill the gap in information on race, ethnicity and mental health, but differences in research design and methodology have made comparability between these studies extremely difficult. Therefore, notwithstanding the uncertainties surrounding the diagnosis and aetiology of psychiatric categories in general, it is heavily problematic making any confident generalizations about the racial and ethnic composition of those in mental distress in Britain. Nevertheless, the evidence available suggests that members of black and ethnic minority groups are frequently over-, under- or mis-diagnosed as mentally ill (Wilson, 1993). However, these probabilities are distributed unevenly among the different groups and diagnostic categories. For example:

- *African-Caribbean People* are more likely than their white British counterparts to be diagnosed as suffering from schizophrenia and less likely to be diagnosed as suffering from depression (Cochrane, 1977; Dean *et al.*, 1981; Harrison *et al.*, 1988; Littlewood and

Lipsedge, 1987; Thomas *et al.*, 1993); admitted to hospital, on a compulsory order, and with the involvement of the police (Carpenter and Brockington, 1980; Cope, 1989; Dean *et al.*, 1981; Ineichen, 1986; Ineichen *et al.*, 1984; McGovern and Cope, 1987; Pinto, 1970; Rogers and Faulkner, 1987; Rwgellera, 1977); detained in more secure settings (Bolton, 1984; Cope, 1989); and treated with medication and ECT rather than with psychotherapy (Bolton, 1984; Bryan *et al.*, 1985; Littlewood and Cross, 1980).

- *Asian People* in Britain are more likely to be diagnosed with depression (Beliappa, 1991) and to a lesser extent schizophrenia (Carpenter and Brockington, 1980; Hitch, 1981); admitted to hospital under an emergency order, and are reluctant to use preventative mental health services (Webb-Johnson, 1991).
- *Irish People* in Britain are grossly over-represented as users of psychiatric services (Bracken *et al.*, 1998; Greenslade, 1994). They have the highest rates of mental hospitalization and are over-represented in most diagnostic categories (Cochrane, 1977; Cochrane and Bal, 1989). Irish rates of schizophrenia are second only to those of the African-Caribbean population.

Moreover, there is very little research data on the experiences of other significant minority groups such as the Jewish, Somali and Chinese communities in Britain.

Francis (1989) suggests that the question of race and ethnicity is not just another discrete demographic factor that can be understood within a positivistic, medical model of cause and effect. Rather it is an issue that questions psychiatry's role and function within society. To this end, critical researchers and writers have sought first, to question whether these racialized divisions reflect genuine differences in rates of mental distress between ethnic groups. Are they the result of some innate biological or psychological vulnerability; exposure to environmental stress; or are they the consequences of fundamentally flawed diagnostic frameworks and professional practices? Second, there has been a commitment to documenting the experiences of black and ethnic minority individuals and groups in the mental health system. Unfortunately most of these experiences reflect patterns of overt and institutional racism – whether intentional or unintentional. Such accounts have challenged medical psychiatry and the mental health system to listen and respond to the expressed views and needs of these service users. This has resulted in some positive initiatives, though the reality is that racism is both pervasive and persistent.

Chakrabarti defines racism as:

A set of beliefs or a way of thinking within which groups identi-fied on the basis of real or imagined biological characteristics (skin colour, for example) are thought necessarily to possess other characteristics that are viewed in a negative light. It is rooted in the belief that certain groups, identified as 'races', 'ethnic minori-ties' or by some more abusive label, share characteristics such as attitudes or abilities and a propensity to certain behaviour. The assumption is made that every person, whether man, woman or child, classified as belonging to such a group is possessed of all these characteristics.

(1990: 15)

This definition clearly includes a number of key elements:

- Beliefs and values are a part of racism; that is racism is an ideology.
- It relates to 'real or imagined biological characteristics'. Racism is therefore socially constructed rather than biologically given.
- Racism is a negative term: it has strong negative connotations and is used as a form of abuse (and, by extension, discrimination and oppression).
- Stereotypical assumptions are used to sustain this negativity and thus maintain the dominance, power and privilege of the white majority.

(Thompson, 1993: 60)

Bracken *et al.* (1998: 105) argue that it is important to move beyond categorizations of race and ethnicity purely in terms of skin colour since they 'are simply inadequate to address the complex ethnic reality of modern Britain'.

Racism and mental health are connected in several important respects:

- In definitions of mental health and illness.
- In theories of causation.
- In assessment and diagnosis.
- In the services and treatments provided.
- In the organizations and institutions which make up the mental health system.
- In the training of mental health professionals.

These connections also articulate with each other in significant ways.

Definitions of mental health and illness

The dominant theme in Western culture is that problems to do with a person's emotional life are conceptualized as illnesses that require the intervention of trained 'experts' – psychiatrists and psychologists. Since the nineteenth century, mental health problems have been constructed and responded to within a predominantly medical framework (see Chapter 1). The processes involved in defining, identifying, explaining and responding to such problems have been governed by a subscription to an ever-expanding array of illness categories that draw spurious boundaries around 'normality' and 'abnormality'. Although there are many variations of the basic illness model incorporating biological, psychological and social factors, they all share an ability to bestow on a professional group the power to decide what constitutes 'madness', who is 'mad' and how they should be treated. Moreover, in spite of claims to scientific neutrality, these processes have been found to be profoundly influenced by historical, cultural, ideological, socio-economic and political contingencies.

Suman Fernando (1988, 1995) argues that the values, ideologies and assumptions of Western European culture have fashioned and permeated psychiatry so that, from a non-Western viewpoint, the illness model of mental health is alien and alienating. For example, generally speaking, the Western notion of a strict division between mind and body (Cartesian dualism) is at odds with Eastern thinking which emphasizes a holistic approach to health and well-being. Moreover, the ideals for mental health differ considerably:

> In Eastern thinking integration, balance and harmony, both within oneself and within the family or community, are important aspects of what may be considered mental health, while in the West, self-sufficiency, efficiency and individual autonomy seem to be important.
>
> (Fernando, 1995: 17/18)

Although racism has existed for centuries, racist stereotypes worked their way into the fabric of mental health theory and practice from the nineteenth century onwards:

> As psychiatry and psychology confronted other cultures and races, ideologies within the disciplines reflected to a greater or lesser extent Western thinking about black, brown, yellow and red

people (so called). Their 'mind', and hence their propensity to illness of the mind, was identified as inherently different to that of white people.

(Fernando, 1995: 39)

Not only were their minds considered different, but also inferior to those of whites. Many of these stereotypes originate in the era of colonialism and slavery. For example, some highly influential early psychologists and psychiatrists (such as Freud, 1913; Maudsley, 1867; Pritchard, 1835; and Tuke, 1858) subscribed to the idea that non-Europeans were 'savages' with primitive instincts and therefore no capacity for mental illness. Others claimed black people had an 'instinct for submission' (McDougall, 1920) and as slaves 'become prey to mental illness when set free' (Cartwright, 1851) (all cited in Fernando, 1992). Such stereotypes have their modern equivalents, for example in the perception of African-Caribbean service users as potentially violent and dangerous; of Asians as 'passive' people who 'look after their own'; the construction and application of diagnoses such as 'ganja psychosis' to African-Caribbeans; or in assumptions that black people are linguistically or intellectually incapable of benefiting from psychotherapy.

Theories of causation

On the basis of these observations it is of no surprise to find that racism is implicated in the formulation of theories of mental health and illness. As already stated, such theories encompass biological, psychological and socio-cultural explanations. Western mental health research has focused primarily on the hypothesis that mental disorder has a biological basis expressed in terms of a mixture of genetic, biochemical and brain abnormalities. However, as yet, decades of expensive bio-medical research has failed to produce unequivocal evidence to support such claims. There remains a substantial degree of uncertainty surrounding this whole area (Barnes, 1987; Bentall, 1992; Jenner *et al.*, 1993; Lieberman and Koreen, 1993).

Errol Francis (1991: 82) notes how 'the oldest and most enduring explanation of perceived differences in psychiatric morbidity according to race is that there are genetic differences in susceptibility to mental illness'. The classical arguments of social Darwinism have been conflated with theories about genetic predisposition to conditions such as schizophrenia, representing a potent blend of ideology and science. Pilgrim and Rogers note:

The link between race and mental illness has historically been a close one and medical-scientific knowledge has been far from neutral about the assumed relationship. It has played a significant role in the perpetuation of pejorative theories and oppressive practices about certain groups.

(1993: 46)

Although biological theories of racial difference were somewhat discredited in the wake of the Nazi holocaust, the bio-medical approach has remained dominant in the conceptualization and treatment of mental distress throughout the twentieth century. Indeed bio-genetic arguments have acquired a renewed confidence in work which has reinvigorated notions of biological and racial inferiority (Herrnstein and Murray, 1994; Rushton, 1988, 1990). Beardsley highlights the all too familiar political and ideological overtones in such work:

The arguments stem from the same tradition of biological determinism that led, not so long ago, to compulsory sterilizations in the USA and genocide elsewhere.

(in Harris, 1995: 5)

This is not to suggest that anyone subscribing to biological theories of mental distress is inherently guilty of subscribing to racist notions of inferiority and superiority. Such notions become relevant only when those doing the theorizing add the assumption that a particular racial group exhibits a greater biological predisposition to mental distress than other racial groups. However, as Fernando (1991: 22) states 'although the biological differentiation of people on the basis of race has been exploded as a myth, the reality of race as a social marker persists in association with the persistence of racism'.

Socio-cultural factors have also been influential as explanations for the apparent differences in the occurrence of mental distress between racial groups. In post-war Britain cultural difference began to be emphasized as a basis for identifying black and ethnic minorities as 'out-groups' (Husband, 1994). A belief in the biological inferiority of black and ethnic minorities was no longer necessary to justify their exclusion (Barker, 1981). Gilroy (1993: 23) notes that British racism now 'frequently operates without any overt reference to "race" itself or the biological notions of difference which still give the term its common-sense meaning'. Although this 'new racism' plays down the significance of biological difference, it is still discriminatory and 'deficit'-focused insofar as it emphasizes *cultural* difference. Dominelli

(1988) argues that both 'new' and 'old' racism serve to pathologize black and ethnic minority individuals and families – to present them as inferior to their white British counterparts. Francis (1991: 83) notes how black and ethnic minority cultures 'have been variously theorized as weak, bastardized and unstable, giving rise to acculturated, unstable families and deviant individuals'.

Other perspectives have looked to psychological problems associated with acculturation to white British society, producing 'culture shock', 'identity crisis' and 'trans-generational conflict' (Littlewood and Lipsedge, 1998). The implication is that black and ethnic minority people, even when born in Britain, have an innate difficulty with psychological change and cultural adjustment. Such theories have been accused of being culturally reductionist, of victim-blaming, and of failing to confront the reality and complexity of racism in the lives of black and ethnic minority people in Britain (Burke, 1984; Donovan, 1986; Fernando, 1986; Mercer, 1986). This has led to a debate between 'transculturalists' and 'anti-racists' in mental health theory and practice. The former argue for the recognition of cultural diversity (Ballard, 1979; Littlewood and Lipsedge, 1998; Rack, 1982) while the latter are more concerned with challenging the power of white psychiatry (Fernando, 1988; Mercer, 1986). Anti-racist perspectives emphasize the impact of structural oppression – poverty, racial harassment, discrimination in education, employment, housing, health – on the mental health of black and ethnic minority people (Beliappa, 1991; Fenton and Sadiq, 1991). They also draw on social constructionist perspectives to argue that black people's resistance to oppression has been pathologized as mental illness (Mercer, 1986).

Fernando suggests that highlighting the significance of racism in mental health theory and practice is not to deny the relevance of culture. Cultural differences in the expression of distress; in concepts of 'health' and 'illness'; and in expectations of helping agencies all need to be acknowledged and responded to, but in such a way that does not perpetuate and reinforce inaccurate stereotypes. He states:

> An emphasis on culture, however well-intentioned, may lead to a racist approach in practice ... the promotion of cultural sensitivity without challenging racism may result in the reinforcement of racism by masking it and thereby inducing complacency.
>
> (1988: 167)

The potency of stereotypes derives from the fact that they are much more than misrepresentations. Following the work of Fanon (1967,

1986), Fernando (1988: 30) explains how 'stereotypes are, to a large extent, the medium for political manipulation and the exercise of (racist) power'. Fanon illustrates how life within a colonial situation influences the personalities of those colonized. Through the experience of being treated as an inferior human being in one's own country, black people often internalize the negative stereotypes held of them by white society, and in so doing help to maintain their own oppression. Such a negative identity needs to be challenged, confronted and changed through interventions which promote ethnic pride, identity and thereby self-esteem. Fanon's analysis has been extended to the situation of black and ethnic minorities living in Britain through the development of projects which encompass both individual psychotherapy and collective 'conscientization' (Holland, 1990; Sashidharan, 1986) reflecting the idea that black people needed to redefine themselves by asserting their own history and culture.

Assessment and diagnosis

The development and refinement of intricate classification and diagnostic systems such as the Diagnostic and Statistical Manual of the American Psychiatric Association (APA, 1994) and the International Classification of Diseases of the World Health Organization (WHO, 1992) were intended to eradicate subjective bias in diagnostic practice. However, research has revealed the persistence of negative cultural stereotyping. In their study of 290 psychiatrists, Loring and Powell (1988: 1) found that the 'sex and race of client and psychiatrist influence diagnosis even when clear cut diagnostic criteria are presented'. The psychiatrists ascribed violence, suspiciousness and dangerousness to black clients, with black males being more likely to be diagnosed as paranoid schizophrenic and both black males and females being more likely to be diagnosed as having a paranoid personality disorder. Loring and Powell (1988: 19) conclude, 'even with carefully drawn standards, diagnosis will remain a subjective activity'. This trend is confirmed in other studies. For example, Lewis *et al.* (1990) found psychiatrists' perceptions of patients, the type and severity of diagnosis, and the type of treatment offered, were all affected by the factor of race.

Some suggest that ethnocentric bias in diagnostic practice leads to the misattribution of psychiatric labels to non-Western people (Fernando, 1988; Littlewood and Lipsedge, 1998). Accordingly, labels such as 'schizophrenia' and 'cannabis psychosis' are misapplied to the disturbed behaviour of African-Caribbean people, and labels such as depression are under-used. However, this view has been criticized by those who would argue that it does not go far enough in challenging the validity of the diagnostic categories or practices *per se* (Sashidharan, 1986). These critics suggest that 'race and culture are inextricably bound up in the construction of disease categories' (Pilgrim and Rogers, 1993: 55) and that it is the use of fundamentally flawed diagnostic criteria that has led to invalid conclusions concerning the nature and degree of mental distress in black and ethnic minority populations.

Treatment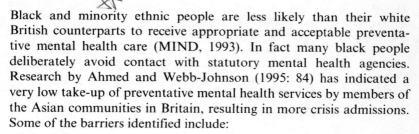

Black and minority ethnic people are less likely than their white British counterparts to receive appropriate and acceptable preventative mental health care (MIND, 1993). In fact many black people deliberately avoid contact with statutory mental health agencies. Research by Ahmed and Webb-Johnson (1995: 84) has indicated a very low take-up of preventative mental health services by members of the Asian communities in Britain, resulting in more crisis admissions. Some of the barriers identified include:

- Lack of awareness of existing services.
- Lack of awareness of what services can offer.
- Language and communication barriers.
- Lack of appropriate and accessible information about existing services.
- Lack of confidence in the ability of services to understand and meet needs.
- Perception of services as not user-friendly.
- Fear that confidentiality will not be preserved.
- Negative past experiences of services.

The majority of people who enter psychiatric care do so as informal patients, although the extent to which this represents genuine choice or familial/professional pressure and persuasion is a matter of debate. However, this is not the case for certain members of black and ethnic minority communities who are more likely to be referred to hospital under the compulsory procedures of the 1983 *Mental Health Act* (Cope, 1989; Littlewood and Lipsedge, 1998; Moodley and Perkins, 1991; Pipe *et al.*, 1991). Browne (1995: 67) points to 'the way in which the thread of perceived dangerousness of black individuals runs through the civil sectioning process'.

Once in hospital, black and ethnic minority patients, particularly African-Caribbeans, are over-represented in locked wards and secure units (Bolton, 1984; Jones and Berry, 1986). They are also more likely to receive the harsher forms of psychiatric treatment, including large doses of neuroleptic medication and ECT (Bolton, 1984; Chen *et al.*, 1991; Littlewood and Cross, 1980; Shaikh, 1985). They also have less access to talking therapies (MIND, 1993). The line between 'treatment' and 'control' can become dangerously blurred, as seen in the case of Orville Blackwood who died in Broadmoor hospital in 1991 after receiving excessive doses of major tranquillizers (Prins *et al.*, 1993). This is all the more significant since in 1989 the Mental Health Act Commission had drawn attention to and expressed concern about the high level of medication administered to African-Caribbean patients. MIND (*The Guardian*, 27 August 1994) estimates that one death a week can be attributed to neuroleptic medication and many of these cases involve black people. These deaths go largely unnoticed in the clamour around media-induced panics about 'dangerous' psychiatric patients 'freed to kill in the community' (Schizophrenia Media Agency, 1995).

The mental health system

Not only has research revealed discriminatory practices in the provision of mental health services to different ethnic groups in Britain, but also in the employment of black people within health and welfare services (Bryan *et al.*, 1985; Dominelli, 1988; Donovan, 1986; Doyal, 1979; Rooney, 1987; Torkington, 1983, 1991). Racism manifests itself in a number of ways in contemporary health and welfare organizations – 'it may appear overtly in *personal* forms; it may be *institutionalized* in organizational structures and practices; and it may be seen in the framework of *policies* for the caring professions' (Hugman, 1991: 149). This has led to a range of responses, in particular the development of equal opportunities policies. However, there have been criticisms that such strategies fail to acknowledge the centrality of racism as the key issue rather than the notion of 'opportunity' (Hugman, 1991). Owusu-Bempah (1989) suggests that equal opportunities statements can be used as a smokescreen which obscures the pervasiveness of structural racism. Thus it is argued that for any progress to be made, anti-racist strategies must be developed. An anti-racist approach acknowledges the links between race and other forms of oppression or exclusion and is therefore geared towards addressing the complex, multi-faceted nature of oppression. As Hugman (1991: 159) notes, 'without this emphasis policies remain trapped at the level of ideal intentions because they can be subverted, opposed or can produce unintended consequences'.

Training of mental health professionals

There has been extensive criticism of traditional approaches to education and training of health and welfare personnel (Dominelli, 1988). However, recently there have been more positive developments in the field of race equality training. Ferns and Madden (1995: 108) define race equality training as 'promoting race equality in a productive and creative way, adapted to the needs of individual participants in the training, so that they go away able to tackle both personal discrimination as well as institutional racism'. The main focus is on identifying patterns of institutional racism; removing barriers to race equality and creating accessible and appropriate services for black and ethnic minority users. They highlight the following features:

* Raising awareness of institutional and personal racism.
* Analysing service provision from a race equality perspective.
* Constructive criticism of professional practice.
* Examining current good practice.
* Empowering of black users and carers.
* Quality of training linked to service improvement.
* User and carer participation in services.
* Action planning to implement race equality.
* Local practical issues addressed.
* Integrated multi-agency approaches reinforced.
* Taking a holistic approach to assessment and service delivery.
* Your personal responsibility for race equality emphasized.

Ferns and Madden suggest it is important to develop a broad strategic approach to race equality training in order to avoid it becoming tokenistic. To this end training should always be linked with policy development to ensure the transition from words to action.

Clearly there is now a wide body of evidence from critical research which suggests that mainstream mental health services have both failed to provide appropriate services for black and ethnic minority communities and also to consult effectively with such communities in determining what types of services they need. Even the conservative NHS Mental Health Task Force has admitted that:

> Predominant psychiatric treatment does not take account of the impact of race and racism. Likewise, there is no widespread acceptance of the importance of culturally diverse methods in working with Black mental health service users and carers.
>
> (cited in Jennings, 1996: 1)

Innovations in practice: the voluntary sector

It has primarily been agencies in the voluntary sector which have attempted to fill the gap in mainstream mental health services. These are usually on the margins of health and social care provision and are generally modest, small-scale, local initiatives such as:

- *The African-Caribbean Mental Health Association* – which provides counselling, legal representation, housing and befriending schemes in Brixton, London.
- *The Fanon Project* – which provides a day centre for African-Caribbean people in London.
- *Shanti* – a counselling service for black women by black counsellors in South London.
- *Nafsiyat* – which provides psychotherapy services for black and ethnic minority clients in London.
- *Harambee* – which provides support and accommodation for single homeless black people with mental health problems in Handsworth, Birmingham.
- *The Mental Health Shop* – which offers advice, information and support to people experiencing mental health problems and their carers in Leicester.

However, the trend towards marketization of health and welfare services, brought about by the introduction of the 1988 *Local Government Act* and the 1990 *NHS and Community Care Act*, has led to substantial changes in the character and function of many of these initiatives (Haughton and Sawa, 1993; Latimer, 1992; Wenham, 1993). Local authorities are no longer the main providers of services but 'enablers', so that increasingly 'the voluntary sector is being incorporated into the state's commercial delivery mechanism for purchasing care from the cheapest provider' (Ahmed and Webb-Johnson, 1995: 73). Ahmed and Webb-Johnson note how these changes have the potential to undermine the traditions of innovation and vibrancy in the voluntary sector since the provision of grants to voluntary agencies has been replaced by a system of compulsory competitive tendering. Additionally, the traditional roles of advocacy and campaigning are in danger of being eroded. Ironically therefore, although these services have been identified as responsive to the needs of their communities (Ahmed and Webb-Johnson, 1995; Hinds, 1992) they operate under precarious conditions *vis-à-vis* staffing and resources.

Innovations in practice: the statutory sector

It is widely acknowledged that the traditional structure of mental health service provision has been somewhat rigid and inflexible. This has meant that many people in mental distress, particularly from the black and ethnic minority communities, have encountered statutory services which are inappropriate to their needs 'because they do not "fit" the service based on traditional models of "illness" and treatment' (Moodley, 1995: 121). Moodley argues that a good mental health system should 'provide services that fit the clients rather than ones that force the clients into a predetermined mould'. She outlines the work of *The Maudsley Outreach Support and Treatment Team (MOST)* as a good example of an accessible, acceptable and appropriate outreach service within the statutory sector. Situated in a shop front on the local high street, the key elements of the service are identified as:

- Priority to people in severe mental distress who are not successfully engaged by services elsewhere.
- Tailor-made treatment plans linked to other community resources and programmes.
- Assertive outreach techniques.
- The development of co-operative, eclectic strategies.
- Responsiveness to local culture, the effects of racism and population needs.

Other good examples are *The White City Mental Health Project – Women's Action for Mental Health* which offers individual psychotherapy and groupwork to all women, and *The Lambo Centre* which offers a day centre to African-Caribbean mental health service users and their carers. Holland (1995: 143) emphasizes the need for more of these small-scale, innovative projects to 'fight their way into the mainstream' in order to ensure progressive multi-ethnic resources in the mental health system.

Innovations in practice: partnerships

Jennings (1996) notes the trend towards partnerships between statutory and voluntary sector organizations and local communities in planning, developing and implementing better mental health services for black and ethnic minority service users. Such partnerships operate at a variety of levels including:

- General consultation meetings with local communities regarding the development of services.
- Joint planning and policy-making groups.
- Research into the needs of particular groups of users or carers.
- Contracting of service delivery to external agencies.
- Consultation meetings to monitor/evaluate service delivery.
- Joint financing and/or delivery of services.

According to Jennings, the track record for multi-racial partnerships is generally not good. They have been characterized by mistrust and suspicion; worries about the loss of a 'black perspective' or 'selling out'; and a cynicism about the commitment to change. This demonstrates the need for partnership members to have credibility in the black and ethnic minority communities, with an emphasis on openness and power sharing.

The London-based *Sanctuary* projects – *Ipamo,* and *The Hackney African-Caribbean Crisis Centre* – are excellent examples of how such partnerships can succeed. Initiated by the King's Fund Development Centre as an alternative to hospital-based services, the Projects' aims are:

- To provide a community-based crisis support service.
- To provide an acceptable service for the black community which they would use.
- To ensure that the services would become independent, black-managed agencies.

They offer crisis support; short-stay accommodation; respite for families; 24-hour advice/advocacy; counselling and outreach services; and community education. *The Lewisham Black Users and Carers Project* is a similar initiative financed by the King's Fund, Lewisham Social Services, and Lewisham and Guy's Mental Health Trust.

Women and black and ethnic minority people are not unique in experiencing oppression within the mental health system. Their experiences are part of a much wider and long-standing dissatisfaction with psychiatry (discussed in more detail in the following chapter). It is therefore important to recognize the link between the critiques explored in this chapter and the wider critiques of mental health theory and practice that have emerged over the last four decades (Foucault, 1967, 1977; Goffman, 1961; Laing, 1959, 1961, 1967; Scheff, 1966; Scull, 1979, 1981, 1989, 1993; Szasz, 1961, 1963). However, in the context of the current preoccupation with post-modern identities there has been a tendency to see these various critical perspectives in tension with each other and of little relevance. This tendency has the potential to fragment and depoliticize human struggle, establishing hierarchies of oppression. While it is essential to acknowledge difference, this does not negate the fact that there are commonalities and continuities in people's experiences of oppression. Indeed this chapter has highlighted the concrete practical impact of a whole range of contributions. If we look beyond the rhetoric of conflict surrounding critical psychiatry, it is clear that fundamental ideological connections are shared. This means there is a need to emphasize the validity of *all* contributions that aim to improve our understanding of, and response to, the experience of mental distress.

6 Crises of legitimacy

Although the medico-scientific language underpinning psychiatric theory and practice is both powerful and persuasive, beneath this veneer psychiatry is characterized by turbulence and controversy (Busfield, 1996). Its legitimacy has been contested at a variety of levels regarding the boundaries of madness, categorizations of madness, causes of madness and responses to the mad. Moreover, far from being a phenomenon peculiar to the 1960s and 1970s, critiques of psychiatry are as old as the profession itself. Throughout its existence psychiatry has been subjected to radical challenges and resistance from both within and outside its ranks – a reality which has all too often been ignored or dismissed in social histories of the profession. While specific challenges have surfaced at specific historical moments, dissent and resistance to psychiatric authority has been remarkably consistent. In this sense, as Scull (1981) observes, contemporary crises of legitimacy in mental health theory and practice echo earlier such crises confronted by the psychiatric profession. Challenges to psychiatry can be identified at four key sites: theoretical, technological, institutional and legislative (Miller, 1986). Each of these is explored in turn, although it should be recognized that of greater significance is the manner in which they converge and intersect in mental health practice.

The legitimacy of psychiatric knowledge

Contested boundaries of madness: madness as 'illness'

In Western societies, from the second half of the nineteenth century onwards, there was a partial retreat from the primacy of psychological understandings of mental distress in favour of a more somatic model (Fernando, 1988). In the broader context of a burgeoning scientism, there was an increasing acceptance, in both lay and professional terms, that mental problems constituted *illnesses*, just like physical illnesses. The somatic approach appeared to be supported by the discovery of an organic basis to the condition 'general paresis of the insane'. Ironically though, in the context of a strong challenge from within neurology, psychiatry based its nineteenth century professional knowledge claims on the notion that mental disorder was *distinctive* from other illnesses (Busfield, 1986). Therefore, to the extent that it did not and does not draw *exclusively* on the natural sciences, psychiatry has faced an ongoing tension in its relationship with its parent medicine. Nevertheless, the profession consolidated itself in the twentieth century through its assimilation to mainstream medicine, and the concept of 'mental illness' evolved as a generic term, embracing a diversity of behaviours and phenomena. These range from conditions where there is a fairly strong consensus for a biological explanation (such as the dementias) to those where not only is the aetiological evidence less clear cut, but their status as illnesses at all is fiercely disputed (as with schizophrenia).

The debates around schizophrenia in particular illustrate the depth of controversy around the illness model in psychiatry. Although it has probably been the subject of more 'scientific' research than any other category of mental disorder, schizophrenia remains an illusive and highly contested phenomenon. For some time dissenters from within and outside the profession have pointed to the philosophical and methodological flaws inherent in the concept (Bentall, 1992; Boyle, 1993; Ciompi, 1982; Laing, 1959; Szasz, 1961). Ciompi's longitudinal research led him to conclude that 'the concept of schizophrenia lacks validity given the enormous variations in outcomes and life experiences, and the key to understanding "it" lies in making sense of people's individual life patterns' (cited in Ramon, 1996: 55). More recently, the work of Romme and Escher (1993) on voice-hearing has challenged one of the most deeply held assumptions within psychiatry – that hearing voices is a symptom of a disease process and a sure indicator of serious mental illness. This important work suggests that the experience of voice-hearing may be much more common than most psychiatrists believe and may not be limited to the realms of 'abnormal' experience.

The post-modern notion of multiple and conflicting interpretations of reality presents an enormous challenge to a profession so immersed in the modernist enterprise of medicine. Thomas (1997: 241) refers to this as the 'death of certainty'. Such uncertainty does not sit comfortably with many psychiatrists who remain devoted to the biological approach. Indeed, recent developments within sections of the Royal College of Psychiatrists appear to indicate a desire on the part of these stalwarts to distance themselves from the eclectic approach in favour of a closer alliance between psychiatry and neuroscience:

> support of neuroscience in psychiatry will imply a stand against non-scientific discourse. In particular the claims for some anthropological, psychosocial or post-modern 'explanations' in psychiatry appear to reject hypothesis testing as it is commonly understood within the natural sciences. Such approaches are likely only to bring discredit to the intellectual study of psychiatry and further confuse its practice.
>
> (Goodwin cited in Thomas, 1997: 151)

Thomas is highly critical of this tendency amongst some of his peers, seeing it as indicative of 'mindless psychiatry':

> We must allow ourselves to be moved by others. Psychiatry has lost touch with this ability, indeed it is questionable whether it ever possessed it in the first place. Each step into the spurious certainty of neuroscience is a step away from matters of human concern.
>
> (1997: 150)

He is unequivocal about the need for the profession, in the face of the lack of credibility and validity of the illness model, to redefine its ethics in terms of an ethics of inter-subjectivity.

Contested boundaries of madness: madness as 'deviance'

While many psychiatrists argue that mental disorders should be explained and treated as illnesses, sociological theorists and dissident clinicians have tended to draw connections between mental disorder and models of social deviancy (Becker, 1963; Foucault, 1967; Goffman, 1961; Laing, 1967; Scheff, 1966; Szasz, 1961). One of the most controversial disputes in this regard is that between medical psychiatry, the law, and the general public in respect of 'criminal insanity' – the 'mad' or 'bad' debate. The legitimacy of medical psychiatry to arbitrate in decision-making as to whether an offender can be considered responsible in law for his/her actions has been frequently challenged. For example, on two occasions in the early

1980s, in the trials of the mass murderers Peter Sutcliffe (the 'Yorkshire Ripper') and Denis Nilsen, juries disregarded the views of expert psychiatrists that these men were mentally disordered, although the psychiatrists in each case provided evidence of the defendant's diminished responsibility.

More recently, the legitimacy of psychiatry in this area has been contested from a different perspective, in the context of the conviction of Michael Stone in 1998 for the murders of Lin and Megan Russell. During the inevitable post-trial soul-searching for an answer to the question of why and how Stone could commit this appalling act, and how it might have been prevented, it was revealed that he has a long-standing psychiatric diagnosis of 'personality disorder' and an equally long history of violent crime. In this particular case, many have expressed the opinion that psychiatrists and the current mental health legislation are at fault since with the 'untreatable' condition of 'personality disorder' Stone could not be compulsorily detained and was therefore 'allowed' to kill. In the House of Commons the Home Secretary, Jack Straw, launched a verbal attack on psychiatrists, accusing them of washing their hands of 'dangerous psychopaths' (cited in Steele, 1998). In defence of the profession, one anonymous psychiatrist remarked, 'at the moment, no psychiatrist in their right mind would take someone on with a criminal record as they reckon they might end up pilloried by a tribunal or review' (cited in Steele, 1998: 22).

The debate about the legitimacy and/or usefulness of the category of 'psychopathy' or 'anti-social personality disorder', and whether people 'diagnosed' as such should be dealt with within the mental health or criminal justice system, has raged for decades. Critics within and outside the profession have referred to it as a 'dustbin' definition (Prins, 1980). Pilgrim (cited in Steele, 1998: 23), in a letter to Jack Straw, commented that 'conceptually the category has the same logic status as "evil" '. Clearly this presents serious difficulties for psychiatry's credibility insofar as there is so much uncertainty and internal conflict surrounding this subject, yet the profession continues to make expert knowledge claims in respect of such problem behaviour. We will return to this issue later, in the wider context of an analysis of the controversial issue of 'dangerousness' and risk assessment in psychiatry.

Contested boundaries of madness: 'normality' and 'abnormality'

Fernando (1988: 75) argues that the boundary between mental health and mental disorder is concerned with the controversial subject of 'normality'. He cites Sabshin's four approaches to the concept as used by American psychiatrists:

- Normality as health in the absence of illness.
- Normality as an ideal state of mind.
- Normality as the average level of human functioning.
- Normality as a process that is judged by the functioning of individuals over a period of time.

Such distinctions are largely imprecise and ill defined. The cut-off point for the identification of health or illness is essentially an arbitrary exercise that can be seen to change over time and between cultures as ideas about and attitudes towards human behaviours change. Johnstone asks:

> How quiet do you have to be before you can be called withdrawn? How angry is aggressive? How sudden is impulsive? How unusual is delusional? How excited is manic? How miserable is depressed? The answers are to be found not in some special measuring skill imparted during psychiatric training, but in the psychiatrist's and relatives' shared beliefs about how 'normal' people should behave.
>
> (1989: 243)

Similarly, Mechanic (1969) has demonstrated how social and emotional factors have a profound influence on the way in which people present an illness.

During the 1920s and 1930s anthropologists such as Ruth Benedict and Margaret Mead, and sociologists such as Kingsley Davis expressed concerns regarding the social and cultural relativity of psychiatric judgements. These themes were picked up again by those such as Goffman, Laing, Szasz and Scheff during the second half of the twentieth century, in the wider context of a tendency of opposition to psychiatric theory and practice (Busfield, 1996; Sedgwick, 1982). There is a long-standing recognition of the need to re-conceptualize notions of mental health and mental distress in terms of a continuum, rather than simply instituting arbitrary cut-off points. This can be traced back to Freud, who argued that psychiatry was in need of a psychological dimension to counteract the narrowness of its scientific base. As Busfield (1996: 57) notes 'Freudian theorizing emphasises the continuity of mental health and pathology and in so doing facilitates an expansion of therapeutic intervention across the range of mental functioning'. Such an approach potentially allows for the acknowledgement of social and moral judgements about the appropriateness or otherwise of human behaviour; recognizes the significance of individual or social agency; and enables a more flexible, contextual and user-centred approach to the mental health needs of individuals. Indeed, the notion of 'normality' or 'norm' has increasingly been challenged in post-modern and post-structuralist analyses of mental health and mental distress (see, for example, Parker *et al.*, 1995).

Contested categories of madness

Categories of mental disorder have been elaborated upon throughout the twentieth century and formalized into psychiatric classification systems. The two most extensively used are the Diagnostic and Statistical Manual of the American Psychiatric Association (DSM) and the International Classification of Mental and Behavioural Disorders of the World Health Organization (ICD) (APA, 1994; WHO, 1992). These systems are the practical devices by which medical psychiatry arranges and orders the diversity of experiences it deals with (Busfield, 1996). However, despite periodic revisions, they have been far from unproblematic, attracting significant criticism on a variety of levels. First, classification systems are designed to group together objects having a common property, and as such are likely to screen out information relating to the uniqueness of individuals. In this sense, Mirowsky and Ross (1989) suggest that classification and diagnostic systems hinder our understanding of mental health problems since they throw away important information about the individual, which might otherwise have been helpful. Once this happens it is unlikely that such information will be recognized as relevant in the future. This approach clearly reflects the legacy of nineteenth century epidemiology and microbiology and the way in which psychiatry moulded itself on the disease model. Second, as indicated above, classification systems over-emphasize the distinction between 'normal' and 'abnormal' states, failing to recognize human thoughts, feelings and behaviour as richly diverse and better represented as a continuum. Third, there are negative consequences associated with the process of classification and diagnosis. Receiving a psychiatric diagnosis can be an intensely stigmatizing experience:

> We have been thought of, at worst, as subhuman monsters, or at best, as pathetic cripples, who might be able to hold down menial jobs as eke out meagre existences, given constant professional

support. Not only have others thought of us in this stereotyped way, we have believed it of ourselves.

(Chamberlain, 1988: xi)

Finally, although classification and diagnostic systems in the mental health field are modelled on the scientific paradigm, the clinical judgements which follow are not valid objective observations but inferences influenced by attitudes and beliefs (Fernando, 1988). Subjective factors are not eliminated since the process relies on the interpretation of human emotions and behaviour, reflecting a whole range of social, political and cultural biases (Fernando, 1991; Loring and Powell, 1988; Russell, 1995). In this sense, the relatively poor performance of psychiatrists in research trials testing the extent to which any two psychiatrists will reach the same diagnosis when presented with the same 'symptoms' is unsurprising. Guimon notes that:

> (DSM) classifications claim to be atheoretical and to deal with diagnosis on an empirical basis but ... diagnostic bias stems less from any technical limitations which are built into the diagnostic and classificatory systems than from the mind and the biases of the psychiatrist.

(1989: 36–37)

Light (1980) highlights the way in which the experience of learning to diagnose 'mental illness' is profoundly influenced by the social, cultural and political contexts in which psychiatric training takes place. Fernando (1988) points to the dominance of a distinctly Western world-view in psychiatric training and practice. Busfield (1996) notes that the intellectual constructions of psychiatrists and other mental health professionals change over time. Therefore what counts as psychiatric knowledge is always under negotiation and subject to revision. For example, some conditions (such as neurasthenia and hysteria) were once frequently diagnosed but have now virtually disappeared from psychiatric practice, having been declassified. In other cases, the condition is simply reclassified as with the transformation of 'minimal brain dysfunction' (MBD) into 'hyperactivity disorder' (HD) and then into 'attention deficit hyperactivity disorder' (ADHD). Finally, there is the tendency of classification and diagnostic systems to encompass ever-increasing areas of human functioning as constituent of 'disorder'. New categories of disorder have been elaborated to encompass phenomena that previously would not necessarily have been considered the domain of the psychiatrist. For example, following the tragic deaths of the cult leader David Koresh and many of his followers at a siege in Waco, Texas in April 1993, the new category of 'religious or spiritual problem' was introduced in the fourth edition of the DSM (APA, 1994).

Some psychiatrists openly acknowledge the limitations of the diagnostic process:

> There are clear indications that among clinicians patterns of diagnostic assessment are changing. For example, as Leff (1992) indicates, the use of the term schizophrenia is essentially in itself inaccurate and covers a range of heterogeneous conditions, which are themselves difficult to define clearly.
>
> (McCrone and Strathdee cited in Ramon, 1996: 5)

In this sense it is hardly surprising that Pilgrim and Rogers (1993: 97) ask the question 'how do mental health professionals with such a weak, controversial, contradictory and poorly credible body of knowledge continue to maintain a mandate to regulate the lives of those they deem to be mentally unfit?'.

The legitimacy of psychiatric technologies

One of the most important consequences of the power of psychiatric theory is that it determines how people with mental health problems are responded to. Throughout the history of psychiatry it has been possible to identify preferences in the approach to psychiatric treatment. While it is true that at any given time certain approaches to treatment pre-dominate, these often co-exist with lesser-used alternatives (Pilgrim and Rogers, 1993). Johnstone (1989: 197–198) suggests that physical treatments in psychiatry all tend to go through predictable cycles of opinion:

1 The initial discovery is accidental.
2 The treatment is greeted enthusiastically.
3 It soon becomes apparent that the treatment is not as effective as first claimed, but it nevertheless becomes one of psychiatry's standard tools.
4 Evidence mounts concerning the treatment's limitations or even its harmful effects.

5   The treatment is abandoned.
6   The cycle begins again with another discovery.

However, irrespective of the vagaries of fashionable therapeutic trends, there is an overriding unresolved tension between those psychiatric technologies that are primarily directed at the body and those which focus on the mind.

Physical treatments

Although moral treatment continued to be a minor part of the psychiatric discourse, the medicalization of madness in the nineteenth century involved a predominantly somatic emphasis. If madness was located in the body, then the logical conclusion was that approaches to its treatment should focus on the body. A typical method used was *restraint* – the use of chains, shackles, leg irons, locked boots, hand/wrist straps, muzzles, strait-jackets, bed straps and restraining chairs. One of the most vivid descriptions of nineteenth century 'treatment' methods can be found in the narrative of John Perceval – a survivor of the early public asylum system. His account of his experiences of restraint offers a valuable insight:

> (my) arms were tied down to each side of the bed by bands of ticking. Still, I continued to excite alarm and, subsequently, my feet were fastened to the bottom of the bed in the leather anklets I had on in the daytime. Fastened thus, lying on my back, I passed my wretched sleepless nights for nearly, if not quite, nine months! To add to my feverishness and misery, the servant usually tied my right arm so tight, passing the thong twice around it, that it cut my flesh, causing a red ring round the arm in the morning.
>
> (in Bateson, 1962: 90–91)

Fennell (1996) argues that a key factor enabling the medical profession to gain a dominant position in the treatment of mental disorder was the 'abolition' of mechanical restraint by the 1870s and the increasing use of chemical restraint. The role of drugs in the treatment of mental disorder at this time was fairly limited and largely restricted to the administration of sedatives such as chloral hydrate, bromides, morphine and paraldehyde. Perceval (in Bateson, 1962: 39) spoke of 'the most filthy medicine that tasted like steel filings in a strong acid'.

Other approaches included *bleeding, vomiting and purging*. These methods were used extensively by physicians in the treatment of all sorts of ailments, not only madness. Again, Perceval's account of his experiences is sobering:

> In my delusions I twice required two severe operations, or was supposed to require; one, bleeding at the temporal artery; the other, having my ear cut open to let out extravasated blood. I had no warning of either of these operations; only, I knew of the second by having some jam with a strong garlic-like medicine brought to me on a piece of bread – which I had given to me once before, the morning before I had my artery cut; that day I was bled till I fainted! I saw my blood taken away in basins full, and I did not know what to anticipate.
>
> (1838/40: 23–24)

Patients might also have been subjected to *water therapy*. This included warm baths, cold baths, vapour baths and water-shock. Perceval describes how he was:

> Occasionally seized hand and foot by two men and thrown suddenly backwards into the bath and I did not know what need there was for violence for I never hesitated to enter it. On one occasion Simplicity stretched out an iron bar to duck my head under the water by pressing it upon my neck; for the men seemed to think it an essential part of their extraordinary quackery to have the head well soused.
>
> (cited in Bateson, 1962: 76–77)

Although there were some significant advances in psychological approaches during the first quarter of the twentieth century (see Chapter 2), by the 1930s there was a revived interest in biological psychiatry which fuelled a wave of experimentation with radical physical treatments. By the late 1930s, psychiatrists were regularly inducing comas, administering electroshocks and performing psychosurgery. Fennell (1996) suggests that this period paved the way for the pharmacological revolution of the 1950s, as it reinforced an experimental ethos and radical pioneering spirit. The risks associated with these radical treatments were played down and overshadowed by the mood of scientific optimism. While psychosurgery is rarely practised nowadays, some clinicians consider electro-convulsive therapy (ECT) to be an effective and ethical treatment. Thus it is still routinely practised in British psychiatric hospitals. This is despite widely reported damaging side effects and the absence of any scientific evidence explaining how it works (Breggin, 1979; Masson, 1990).

Since the mid-1950s, the dominant approach to the treatment of mental distress has been pharmacological. The majority of those diagnosed as mentally ill are treated with powerful psychoactive medication. Moreover, the likelihood of being treated with drugs is increased if the person is working class (Mollica and Mills, 1986), female (Cooperstock, 1981; Ettore and Riska, 1993; Miles, 1988; Penfold and Walker, 1984) or black (Littlewood and Cross, 1980). Drugs are quick and relatively simple to administer in comparison with psychosocial interventions, so it is perhaps unsurprising to find over-reliance on and over-use of medication by GPs and psychiatrists. Pilgrim and Rogers (1993) note that all physical treatments, especially pharmacological treatments, are legitimated and encouraged by the profit motive. Many drug companies not only profit from the sale of psychoactive medication, but also from the production and sale of drugs designed to counter their negative side effects. Similarly, Healy (1990a, 1990b, 1991) has questioned the scientific and objective basis of much psychopharmacological research. He exposes the extent to which commercial interests dominate what is romantically believed to be a domain devoted to scientific discovery in the interests of the 'sick' or disabled.

Nevertheless, there is now more evidence of the limitations and potentially harmful effects of drug treatments. They have been accused of producing 'iatrogenic' effects – that is a tendency to produce new forms of sickness in the very individuals they aim to 'cure' (Illich, 1975, 1976). This can be illustrated with particular reference to the use of minor and major tranquillizers in psychiatry.

The psychopharmacological approach to mental distress from the 1950s onwards created high expectations of and demand for a 'magic bullet' to eliminate emotional distress. The benzodiazepine minor tranquillizers were hailed as a major advance in the treatment of neurosis. Many GPs, so often hard-pressed for time, welcomed the 'quick fix' promised by the drug companies, ignorant of the scale of iatrogenic addiction that was to follow. Although benzodiazepines can be effective in controlling anxiety when prescribed for a short period (*circa* seven to ten days), beyond this they are highly addictive and patients are at risk of severe withdrawal symptoms. These include panic attacks, sleep disturbances, uncontrollable shaking, palpitations, sweating and muscle tension:

I would feel myself becoming very weak and it even affected my voice. I would shake and my heart would beat so fast that sleep was impossible. I felt like my whole insides were shaking and some mornings I had to be sick I felt so ill, for months. I laid about feeling so ill ... If I did fall asleep I would wake up, because my whole body kept jerking. I felt so ill that all I did was cry, it really was hell.

(in Lacey and Woodward, 1985: 63)

Benzodiazepine prescriptions peaked in Britain in 1979 when some 30.7 million scripts were dispensed (Taylor, 1987). Research by Lacey and Woodward in 1985 revealed that one in four British adults had been prescribed benzodiazepines and the majority of these were women. Twenty-five per cent had been prescribed them for more than four months, and some for ten or twenty years. Many GPs and psychiatrists subsequently changed their prescribing habits, however to a great extent the damage had already been done. Significant numbers of people have been struggling with long-term addiction problems, with little or no support from the mainstream mental health services. A variety of self-help organizations such as TRANX, Release and the Council for Involuntary Tranquilliser Addiction emerged to fill the gap and in many instances became focal points for popular protest and collective demands for justice through the legal system. What transpired was the largest class action in British legal history – 17,000 claimants and 2,000 firms of solicitors (Dyer, 1994). However, it collapsed in 1994 when legal aid was withdrawn.

Research studies have generally concluded that neuroleptic medication is effective in helping to control the acute symptoms associated with severe mental illness and may also help to maintain social functioning if taken regularly (Wyatt, 1991). However, as Thomas (1997) notes, many people do not find such medication helpful, nor do all researchers support the assertion that its long-term use improves social functioning (Kane and Freeman, 1994; Schooler, 1991). A good indication of users' experiences of major tranquillizers is reported in Rogers *et al.* (1993). Although 57 per cent of respondents in this study commented that they found medication 'helpful', this was counterbalanced by the fact that more than 60 per cent described 'severe' or 'very severe' side effects.

Acute movement disorders that closely resemble Parkinson's disease may appear soon after starting neuroleptic medication. They are characterized by a general slowing down in movement and responsiveness to the environment, accompanied by tremor, writhing movements and a 'zombie-like' expression. Patients may also experience a drug-induced agitation and depression – a condition referred to as *akathesia*. This is characterized by a severe restlessness and inability to keep still and accounts for much of the 'pacing' behaviour observed on psychiatric wards. Some researchers have noted that these side effects are so distressing that they may be implicated in the high suicide rate among those diagnosed with severe mental illness (Drake and Ehrlich, 1985). Additionally, neuroleptic medication has been found to induce apathy and disinterest in patients – something of an irony given that such behaviour is also considered to be a negative symptom of severe mental illness!

The most disabling long-term side effect is *tardive dyskinesia* – a neurological disorder that can emerge after years of prolonged exposure to major tranquillizers. Patients develop involuntary movements of the jaw, tongue, lips and face. These may not become apparent until medication is reduced or stopped and may disappear when the original dosage is resumed or increased. These side effects are extremely difficult to treat once established and are generally irreversible (Breggin, 1993; Thomas, 1997). These bizarre uncontrollable mannerisms are intensely stigmatizing as to the lay person they have come to epitomize mad behaviour. The following description of the effect of major tranquillizers from a service user illustrates the point:

> Your tongue becomes gross in your mouth, your body twists and many patients are viewed by their families when they come into hospital with these terrible side effects, and it's interpreted as being a facet of their mental condition … and will always be so because nobody ever explains.
>
> (Survivors Speak Out, 1986)

In spite of these adverse consequences, psychiatrists have generally failed to exercise caution in prescribing neuroleptic medication. Thomas (1997) expresses concern that there has been a trend towards prescribing higher doses of medication, often in dangerous combinations, at the substantial risk of sudden death. MIND (*The Guardian*, 27 August 1994) estimate that one death a week is caused by powerful tranquillizers. Of particular concern is the use of such powerful medication as a management tool where heavier sedation makes a patient easier to manage. Even more alarming is the fact that major tranquillizers are also used either disproportionately and/or inappropriately on certain groups of people such as elders or people with mental disabilities in care establishments, prisoners, and on African-

Caribbean men. The inquiry into the case of Orville Blackwood, who died in Broadmoor in 1991 after receiving large doses of tranquillizing medication, suggested that this case reflected the operation of crude stereotypes of black men as potentially dangerous (Prins *et al.*, 1993).

Brown and Funk (cited in Pilgrim and Rogers, 1993) suggest that it is psychiatry's over-reliance on physical medicine for its status which ultimately accounts for the failure of psychiatrists to change their prescribing habits even though patients complain of the ineffectiveness and/or negative effects of medication. Users report that their views are often ignored or dismissed:

> The psychiatrist said he could help me. I now have a fractured spine through ECT, tardive dyskinesia from their chemicals and I've lost my memory. Many of us who have survived psychiatry know we have been damaged by it. When we complain, we are dismissed as deluded.
>
> (cited in Herman and Green, 1991: 27)

Currently, all patients other than those who are legally compelled under the 1983 *Mental Health Act* have the right to refuse treatment. Before treatment is given they must give legally valid consent to it, and this must be obtained without undue pressure of any kind. Patients must also be given information on the nature and purpose of the treatment, including any serious side effects. Evidence suggests that these conditions are not always adhered to. Cobb (1993) cites a MIND survey that reported 80 per cent of those interviewed thought that they had not been given enough information about their treatment; 84 per cent were not offered a choice of treatments and 52 per cent received a treatment that they did not want. The following accounts from service users are typical:

> I walked into the clinic one day and I was told that they were going to cut my Redeptin injection by half. I am currently on a cocktail of drugs (Lithium, Redeptin and Kemadrin). I was not consulted about this change in medication and I feel that I became ill some months later because of this.
>
> (cited in Clarke, 1994: 59)

> I was threatened with ECT if I did not take Nardil.

> Just told that I was to have anti-depressants and given them – no force but no choice given.

I have just been given treatment. I have neither been asked nor even persuaded. Some of the anti-depressants gave me burning in my throat, which is a very bad side effect. Doctors don't tell you about this.

(cited in Rogers *et al.*, 1993: 166)

Under these circumstances it is not surprising that some patients decide that they do not wish to continue with their medication (Kane and Freeman, 1994). Although psychiatrists often justify their arguments concerning the need for long-term use of medication by referring to the reappearance of symptoms when medication is stopped, it has been argued that this might just as legitimately be attributed to a withdrawal state rather than a true relapse (Thomas, 1997). However, these arguments have tended to go unheard in the debates around community care patients and the 'problem' of drug compliance (Muijen, 1995; Ramon, 1996). In the public imagination the issue appears to be a straightforward one of irresponsibility on the part of certain individuals who are either unwilling or unable to respond positively to the expert advice of clinicians. Such one-sided perceptions of what is a highly complex set of problems have potentially serious consequences for the civil liberties of mental health service users since they have informed the current proposals for legislation to facilitate the compulsory medication of patients in the community (Department of Health, 1998).

Talking treatments

Although there is a clear somatic emphasis in the treatment of mental distress, it has nevertheless been difficult for psychiatry to sustain a purely medical approach. As Ussher (1991: 108) notes 'medicine is not the only voice within orthodox mental health care'. The psychological approaches that emerged in the late nineteenth and early twentieth centuries had a profound influence on the treatment of mental distress. These approaches challenged the legitimacy of the dominant degeneracy theories of insanity, particularly in the context of the 'discovery' of shell-shock during the First World War (see Chapter 2). While the somatic emphasis has remained dominant, the psychological approaches have contributed to the emergence of a more eclectic psychiatry in the twentieth century (Baruch and Treacher, 1978; Treacher and Baruch, 1981).

A variety of activities are encompassed within the term 'talking treatments' ranging from brief supporting discussions with a person who has no formal qualifications, to intensive work over a period of months or even years with a highly trained practitioner. These activities may take place on an individual or group basis, and are broadly based on the notion that through the process of talking, the mentally distressed person may develop an awareness of the source of their distress which may facilitate a return to psychological health. Most professional, paraprofessional or lay helpers have some degree of training in one or more of the orthodox schools of therapy – psychoanalytic, behavioural, cognitive or humanistic (see Chapter 3 for a fuller description of these and other alternative models of therapeutic intervention).

Wood (1993) estimates that some 100,000 people receive talking treatments in Britain. However, due to the fact that NHS provision is severely limited, most of this takes place in the private or voluntary sectors. Clearly in the private sector ability to pay is a major restriction, while in the NHS and voluntary sectors, demand overwhelmingly exceeds supply resulting in long waiting lists. Additionally, black, minority ethnic, working-class, lesbian, gay and older people all have restricted access to talking treatments (Wood, 1993). Research by Lacey and Woodward (1985), Miles (1988), Rogers *et al.* (1993) and Wood (1993) reveals that the demand for talking treatments is most evident amongst people who have been prescribed minor tranquillizers. The service users in these studies related how they really wanted access to someone with whom they could discuss their troubles, but instead were given medication.

Despite the high demand for talking treatments within the mental health system, there are those who have questioned both their efficacy and the extent to which they represent a genuine alternative to the medical approach. Eysenck (1952, 1965) and Rachman (1971) have argued that two-thirds of neurotic patients improve spontaneously regardless of treatment. Others have drawn attention to the 'deterioration effect' in psychotherapy where some patients actually get worse (Bergin, 1971; Bergin and Lambert, 1978). While for some critics the main concern has been to advocate the use of behavioural and/or organic therapies in preference to psychotherapy, for Masson (1990) and Rowe (in Masson, 1990) the key issue is that of the uses and abuses of professional power in psychotherapy. Reflecting on his own training and experiences as a therapist, Masson (1990: 24) suggests that regardless of their good intentions, therapists are 'engaged in acts that are bound to diminish the dignity, autonomy and freedom of the person who comes for help'. He suggests that all therapies (with the possible exception of radical and feminist

\ are self-serving, and demonstrate a lack of interest in social
..e concludes 'what we need are more kindly friends and fewer
professionals' (1990: 30).

Fay Weldon, reflecting on the burgeoning industry in counselling
and psychotherapy observes:

> Therapy, once the much-loved infant saviour, sent among us to
> explain ourselves to ourselves, to make us self-aware, to heal us
> and to cheer us, is in danger of becoming a controlling and rav-
> ening monster.
>
> (1994: 9–10)

Many of the reservations expressed by service users about talking
treatments relate to concerns they have about the abuse of power by
the therapist – emotional, physical and sexual (Rutter, 1995; Wood,
1993). Additionally, it has become evident that talking treatments are
potentially no less open to charges of inherent bias and stereotyping in
relation to class, race, gender, sexuality, disability and age, than any
other mental health intervention (Wood, 1993).

It is clear that, to a greater or lesser extent, all of the main technologies developed and used by psychiatry in the treatment of mental
distress have faced crises of legitimacy – in terms of their lack of
effectiveness, their iatrogenic effects and the ethical issues surrounding
their administration. Furthermore, as Ingelby (1983: 168) observes
'what is conspicuous in this whole field is the almost megalomanic air
of competence and success displayed by the professionals themselves,
in contrast to the intellectual vulnerability of their theories and the
uncertainty of their remedies'. Nevertheless, the uncertainty created by
such crises of legitimacy has facilitated the emergence of new ways of
helping people with mental distress in particular, ways of enabling
people to self-manage their distress. Individuals have always struggled
to develop their own ways of coping. As Herman and Green (1991: 29)
note, 'from the Alleged Lunatics Friends Society of the 1860s to the
Mental Patients Union of the 1960s and early 1970s, there is a tradition
of resistance and of proposing alternatives in the face of a medical
profession and a society seen to be in the grip of fear and ignorance'.

What is different in the contemporary period, however, is the extent
to which new ideas and techniques have been developed and
consolidated in the activities of user groups, sometimes in partnership
with more enlightened mental health professionals:

> The creation of patient-controlled alternatives stands in sharp

contrast to the psychiatric system. Instead of creating clear and stigmatizing distinctions between those who are competent to give help and those who are weak enough to need it, these alternatives are creating new communities of equals, counteracting the alienation and powerlessness most people rightly sense to be a prime cause of their unhappiness.

(Chamberlain, 1988: 113–114)

While there remains a legitimate scepticism that the consumerist emphasis in contemporary mental health service delivery may represent little more than tokenism (Pilgrim, 1993), nevertheless, the momentum towards user-involvement appears unlikely to be halted. As Peter Campbell (in Herman and Green, 1991: 30) states, 'self-advocates will not go back into the closet'.

The legitimacy of psychiatric institutions

During the nineteenth century, a period often characterized as psychiatry's 'golden age', the legitimacy of the profession was challenged most forcefully at the primary site of its activities – the asylum. Even at this early stage the psychiatric institution was identified as predominantly carceral despite its claims to being curative. Once again, the autobiographical accounts of those who experienced psychiatry in these early days offer valuable insights. John Perceval wrote:

I, a nervous patient, was confined in a large room with eleven or more others ... I, weak in body, weak in mind, not able to support fear, or to control it as another, and besides, overwhelmed by superstitious fears. This was my position for six months, until after the hay-making, and then for six months more with the difference of not being tied up. All this was done under the direction of a surgeon, a physician.

(cited in Bateson, 1962: 106)

He continued:

To say that I am surprised at the ignorance of the lunatic doctor would be to say that I am astonished the night should be dark. But how is it that ignorance should so long have been allowed to dupe the world? They seem utterly ignorant of the sufferings of nervous patients.

(cited in Bateson, 1962: 294)

According to Ingelby (1983: 152), although it was the intention of reformers to achieve 'the compulsory public provision and inspection of a nationwide asylum system', they were so keen to achieve their goal that 'they failed to entertain the slightest suspicion that the asylum *itself* might contain severe inherent limitations'. As the populations within the asylums grew (both in terms of overall numbers and in terms of diversity of 'problem'), so too did the criticisms of the institution's ability to function as a medical and curative environment. Increasingly, concern was expressed that the asylum was a tool for maintaining order (Busfield, 1986; Scull, 1993).

During the first half of the twentieth century, the prevention of abuse was not so prominent an issue as it had been in earlier times (Martin, 1984). In the context of an over-optimistic faith in the medical model, the assumption prevailed that the *raison d'être* of hospitals was to do good to their patients. Nevertheless, by the late 1950s, a resurgence of critiques emerged about all aspects of institutional life:

> The common theme of all those who criticised institutions was an abhorrence of the rigid care which ignored human values, dominated by a self-satisfied medical model insensitive to patients' experiences.
>
> (Muijen, 1995: 39)

Miller (1986) delineates three broad lines of institutional critique – therapeutic, political and reformist. The therapeutic lines of institutional critique did not seek to abolish the asylum, but rather to transform it, restoring its curative ideals. The British psychiatrists and psychoanalysts of the Tavistock Clinic (such as Tom Main, Maxwell Jones and their associates) were pioneers in the development of a variety of psychoanalytically based interventions at the Northfield and Mill Hill military hospitals during and after the Second World War. Main gave the name 'therapeutic community' to facilities where the actual setting is designed to promote the psychological treatment of mental distress, although it is Maxwell Jones whose name has primarily become associated with this approach. Pilgrim and Treacher (1992: 19) suggest that 'the British therapeutic community movement became the focus for wide, respectful international interest in democratizing and humanizing the old asylums'.

Of equal significance as a therapeutic line of critique was the work of Russell Barton in the 1950s insofar as it gave formal recognition to the debilitating iatrogenic effects of institutional life. 'Institutional neurosis' was the term Barton used to describe the apathy, loss of initiative and resignation he observed in asylum patients. The importance of Barton's work lay in its revelation of the existence of a relationship between the patient's social environment and their clinical symptoms. However, Barton did not advocate the abolition of the asylum, despite finding such overwhelming evidence of the negative effects of institutional life. Rather, he firmly believed that the adverse effects of institutions could be minimized and patients rehabilitated through the manipulation of their environment and the introduction of progressive and enlightened nursing care (Thomas, 1997).

The enthusiasm around these therapeutic approaches was strongly reminiscent of the moral treatment approach developed at the York Retreat in the nineteenth century. However, as with their predecessors, the achievements of these practitioners were somewhat limited once the tide of professional and public opinion turned against the asylum as an exclusive strategy for the care and treatment of the mentally distressed (Miller, 1986). Nevertheless, the principles and spirit of the therapeutic ideal persists (albeit on a much smaller scale), for example in the work of Richmond Fellowship Hostels, and the Group Homes of the Arbours Association.

The second line of institutional critique can be broadly identified as 'political' insofar as it was principally concerned with the power of the institution. The asylum was criticized in general because of the power it gave society over certain categories of deviant individuals, and in particular because of the power it conferred on the psychiatrist over the patient. Like Goffman (1961), the Italian psychiatrist Franco Basaglia and his associates identified clear parallels between the psychiatric institution and the prison:

> Within its four walls, the pulse of history ceases to beat, the social identity of the individual contained therein is suppressed, and the process of total identification of the individual with its psychic dimensions takes place. The conditions of his life may be offered as proof of his innate inferiority, his culture disregarded as the expression of his irrational deviation. The silence which sets in, in the asylum, becomes both typical of it and guarantees that, from it, no other message will reach the outside world.
>
> (cited in Scheper-Hughes and Lovell, 1987: 275–276)

In contrast to the therapeutic approach, these writers advocated nothing short of the complete dismantling of the asylum. While such a strategy enjoyed some success in the Italian context (culminating in the introduction of legislation phasing out psychiatric hospitals in 1978), in Britain and the USA its impact was far less dramatic. A possible explanation for this is that 'the process central to Basaglia's critical discourse and practice ... is the question of power and empowerment. *All changes came about in a political, not simply technological framework*' (Scheper-Hughes and Lovell, 1987: 45; our emphasis). The transformation of Italian psychiatric practice owed much to the formation of alliances between a 'professional leadership committed to radical change, and organized political and community constituencies from the grassroots level on up'.

The strategy that won ground in Britain and the USA grew out of a distinctively reformist critique of the asylum. Simply this refers to a range of critiques, which have all been concerned with reforming the asylum – both in terms of its nature, size and function, and in terms of its location within the overall mental health system. Miller notes:

> The reformist strategy is strongly critical of the asylum and of its non-curative and even iatrogenic effects. This is undertaken, however, in the name of *another* institutional, administrative and therapeutic apparatus – a new series of sites and practices within which the asylum has a place – albeit one of diminished importance.
>
> (1986: 25)

He suggests that the reformist strategy was firmly 'realist' in its orientation and moderate in its approach. It struck a balance between acknowledging the reality of disempowerment and oppression, but fell short of advocating total abolition and was therefore always much more likely to succeed in the British and American contexts. Such an approach is epitomized in the work of those such as John Wing (1978) and Anthony Clare (1976). Baruch and Treacher (1978) suggest that the reformist strategy facilitated the modernization of psychiatry.

Together, and in various ways, these lines of critique formed the backdrop to the large number of public inquiries into mental institutions from the mid-1960s onwards (Martin, 1984). The patients' experiences in these hospitals were strongly reminiscent of Goffman's (1961) description of total institutions. Martin's (1984: xi) review of these inquiries demonstrates what he refers to as 'the failures of caring in hospitals'. He asks 'how is it that institutions established to care for the sick and helpless can have allowed them to be neglected, treated with callousness and even deliberate cruelty'. Certain recurring features were identified as problematic:

- Isolation of the hospital, wards and staff.
- Lack of support for patients, intensifying their dependency and vulnerability.
- Culture of cruelty as a coping strategy for over-stretched staff.
- The corruption of care where the preservation of order takes precedence over the provision of care.
- Failures of leadership.
- Inadequate/incompetent administration and lay management.
- Inadequate resources and under-staffing.
- Inadequate training.
- Personal failings/corruption.

Even though the attention of these inquiries focused on a relatively small number of hospitals, nevertheless, collectively they demonstrated the failure to acknowledge, let alone resolve, the contradictory discourses of 'care' and 'control' in institutional settings. Moreover, in spite of the inquiries and the subsequent introduction of watchdogs such as the Mental Health Act Commission, the hospital scandals have continued, as for example in the Broadmoor and Ashworth Special Hosptials (Department of Health, 1999; Department of Health/SHSA, 1992; NHS Health Advisory Service/DHSS/SSI, 1988; Prins *et al.*, 1993).

However, it should be noted that while the tone of many accounts of life in psychiatric institutions is overwhelmingly bleak, nevertheless, a number of recent historical contributions have provided a counter-balance to the assumption that all aspects of life in such institutions were negative (Andrews *et al.*, 1997; Broadhurst, 1997; Clark, 1996; Gittins, 1998; Goddard, 1996; Russell, 1997; Valentine, 1996). For example, Diana Gittins (in her research into life in Severalls Hospital in Essex) discovered that the institution had been a thriving and close-knit community, and that many ex-residents had some positive memories:

> Nobody regretted the passing of crowded locked wards, but many felt sad at losing contact with friends and the sense of a refuge set in surroundings where they felt protected from danger and violence.
>
> (Gittins cited in *Community Care*, 21–27 May 1998: 21)

From the late 1980s onwards, the critiques shifted away from an almost exclusive preoccupation with the deficiencies of psychiatric hospitals towards the failures (perceived or actual) of community care legislation, policy and practice (Muijen, 1995). That is, as the sites of psychiatric practice have become more diverse (generally representing a move away from the asylum to the community) so too has the focus of the critique. However, this observation is not as straightforward as it might appear. Up until the early 1980s the inquiries primarily addressed scandals in hospitals on behalf of a public which perceived psychiatric patients as helpless victims of abusive staff and an uncaring insensitive system. By the 1990s, however, the focus and tone of the inquiries changed to reflect a concern with the perceived dangerousness of psychiatric patients living in the community. Since mental health law is predicated to a great extent on the notion of 'danger' (to self and/or others), this shift in focus will be discussed in the wider context of a critique of the legitimacy of mental health legislation.

The legitimacy of mental health legislation

The psychiatric profession has consistently faced challenges to its legitimacy in terms of the legal codification of its activities. Attention has primarily focused on the processes surrounding the detention of individuals identified as mentally disordered, and the supervision and management of psychiatric institutions. Of crucial significance in this has been the creation of a fluid boundary between legal and medical control. Indeed, the tensions and conflicts inherent in the relationship between the two have dominated the history of mental health legislation in England and Wales. At various times since the late eighteenth century legalism has featured strongly in efforts to reform mental health care. From as early as 1763 public interest was aroused concerning the issue of wrongful confinement of individuals in private madhouses (Jones, 1972), and throughout the nineteenth century the psychiatric profession found itself in conflict with a legal profession eager to establish judicial supervision of medical authority (Miller, 1986).

The 1890 *Lunacy Act* has often been cited as the high water mark of legalism in the history of mental health legislation in England and Wales. This legislation empowered the magistracy to arbitrate over petitions for the admission of individuals to asylums and provided for judicial scrutiny of such institutions. However, by the 1920s there was a shift in the focus of concern away from wrongful detention towards the potential harm done to patients by hindering the medical profession in its desire to intervene early in the treatment of the 'mentally ill'. The mood in public policy began to favour the application of preventative social medicine to *both* physical *and* mental illnesses (Jones, 1993). It was argued that the legal requirement of certification was not only a barrier to early treatment but also created fear and stigma around mental illness. Thus, the 1930 *Mental Treatment Act* re-framed public policies for mental health firmly in the language of medicine. It permitted voluntary admission to the newly named 'mental hospitals' and promoted the development of a variety of community-based, non-custodial provisions, free of legal constraints.

This trend towards voluntarism was consolidated in the 1959 *Mental Health Act* which completely abolished judicial involvement in civil proceedings. It framed the powers of the medical profession in the broadest of terms and allowed for a medical judgment as to whether a person was suffering from a mental disorder that warranted detention in hospital. It was argued that this was a progressive move, since the use of compulsory detention would be reserved for the minority of patients and only if it was considered to be in the interests of their health, safety or the protection of others. By the early 1970s more than 80 per cent of admissions to psychiatric hospitals were informal. Rose (1986: 185–186) notes that the 1959 Act 'was part of the general move towards open-door policies within mental hospitals and the integration of psychiatry within the institutions, practices and rationale of general medicine'.

However, once again, during the 1960s, psychiatry came under a barrage of criticism that was largely expressed through debates around rights, liberties and justice. It was suggested that many aspects of psychiatric practice either ignored or openly violated the rights of citizens (Szasz, 1963). In particular, the true 'voluntary' status of patients was fiercely disputed. It was suggested that while it was possible to invoke compulsory legislation for those who refused to be admitted voluntarily, the term was a blatant misnomer. In the British context, many of these criticisms crystallized in a campaign for legal reform spearheaded by MIND in the 1970s. In the review of the 1959 Act that followed, MIND (Gostin, 1975, 1977) pressed for a return to a stronger legalistic framework, arguing that there was an absence of control mechanisms to keep over-zealous psychiatrists in check (although it distanced itself from the overtly libertarian opposition to psychiatry). The new *Mental Health Act* of 1983 generally represented a shift back towards a concern with protecting the individual rights of patients but was limited in its scope to tightening up professional roles and practice only in relation to those patients who were formally detained. To this extent its impact was circumscribed in respect of the experiences of the majority of 'informal' mental health service users (save for the introduction of the Mental Health Act Commission) and it did little for the *collective* rights of patients.

Rose (1986) argues that there are fundamental limitations to rights-based strategies for mental health reform in a society that has no written constitution. Moreover, there are problematic issues to do with competing claims to rights – of the service user, the carer(s), the public etc. Rose suggests that rather than empowering patients, the 1983 legislation merely re-framed and reorganized the power of psychiatry between different forms of professional expertise – medical, legal and social. Additionally, he argues that *rights* strategies have inadvertently contributed to the modernization of psychiatry insofar as they have facilitated 'the relocation of the mental hospital within an expanded psychiatric system' – that is the transfer of the locus of psychiatric control from the hospital to the community (Rose, 1986: 204). It is in the context of the shift from hospital to community-based mental health care that some of the most heated debates have emerged around the legitimacy of psychiatric authority.

The transition from institutional to community mental health care has brought with it many unresolved questions about the nature of mental distress and what constitutes an appropriate response to it. Additionally, a new set of debates and dilemmas has been exposed regarding the management of 'challenging behaviour' and the assessment of risk (Rogers and Pilgrim, 1996). In particular, attention has concentrated on a core group of so-called 'continued care clients' in the community – those with a diagnosis of severe mental illness who have long-term, complex, inter-related difficulties and who for a variety of reasons are considered 'non-compliant'. According to Ramon (1996: 49), this group exposes 'the limitations of the usefulness of psychiatry in both its caring and controlling functions'.

Although it has been established that people with a psychiatric diagnosis make a minimal contribution to violence in society (Department of Health, 1996; Monahan, 1992; Taylor and Gunn, 1999), the issue of 'dangerousness' has recently become a major political issue in the context of wider concerns about the legitimacy of community care legislation, policy and practice. Since the end of 1992 a cluster of tragic incidents (mainly involving individuals with a diagnosis of severe mental illness) have received unprecedented media attention. An impression of widespread, random and irrational danger has been cultivated in the public imagination with headlines such as 'Freed to Kill in the Community' (*Daily Mail*, 2 July 1993). There has been a persistent portrayal of mental health service users as potentially dangerous, violent and unpredictable, or as pathetic victims of their illnesses who should be pitied (Philo, 1996; Philo *et al.*, 1994; Ramon, 1996). The subtext of race is evident in much of this reporting. Francis notes:

> Readers and television viewers are left with subconscious associations between the spectre of unprovoked, inexplicable murder in the street and black psychiatric patients, a potentially explosive combination.
>
> (1996: 4)

Ultimately, such negative stereotyping has served to fuel a moral panic around the perceived dangerousness of mental health service users in the community which has in turn contributed directly to the introduction of repressive policy and legislation, tightening systems of surveillance and control. Since 1 April 1994, NHS mental health service provider units have been obliged to maintain Supervision Registers identifying and providing information on service users 'who are, or are liable to be, at risk of committing serious violence or suicide, or of serious self neglect' (NHS Management Executive, 1994a: 1). On 1 April 1996, the *Mental Health (Patients in the Community) Act 1995* came into force, enabling psychiatrists to order the supervised discharge of certain patients detained in hospital under a section of the 1983 *Mental Health Act*.

For Ramon (1996) such reaction amounts to no less than the demonization of mental health service users. She accuses Marjorie Wallace (the journalist and founder of the pressure group Schizophrenia A National Emergency (SANE)) of irresponsible reporting and sensationalizing the issues around community care. The preoccupation with images of violence and dangerousness has served to distort the process of evaluating the effectiveness of the mental health system in supporting service users in the community. A variety of reports into the care and treatment of those mental health service users involved in the recent tragedies have pointed to inadequacies in the mental health system (Audit Commission, 1994; Blom-Cooper *et al.*, 1995; Department of Health, 1994a, 1994b, 1996; House of Commons Health Select Committee, 1994; Mental Health Foundation, 1994; Nuffield Provincial Hospitals Trust, 1994; Ritchie *et al.*, 1994; Sheppard, 1995). Nevertheless, these structural deficiencies have been overshadowed by the media's amplification of the threat of violence. As Harrison observes, this means that:

> When things go wrong, the fault can be depicted not as inadequate care and services, whether in hospital or the community,

but as the fault of individuals who could *and should* have pre-
dicted and prevented harm, and of the person who should have
complied with the treatment and services they were offered.

(cited in MIND, 1996: 6)

The belief that it is possible to predict and therefore prevent violent
behaviour in individuals with a psychiatric diagnosis has been the
subject of fierce debate for some time. Research in the 1970s
consistently demonstrated the limitations of mental health professionals in assessing 'dangerousness' and current approaches remain
notoriously unreliable (Hopton, 1998; Rogers and Pilgrim, 1996).
Peck concludes:

The assessment of risk and dangerousness is an art not a science,
and a difficult art which requires practitioners to balance past or
present behaviour with predictions of interventions and the civil
liberties of the patient.

(cited in *Community Care*, 9–16 July 1998: 2)

Nevertheless, in the absence of any proven, valid method of assessing
risk, there has been a tendency towards 'playing safe'. The recent
widespread moral panic has meant that psychiatrists are now more
defensive than ever. The enormous public and political pressures
placed on professionals to 'get it right' only serves to distort the
decision-making process and more often than not this is to the
detriment of the patient. For example, one psychiatrist appearing on
the BBC television programme *Panorama* in June 1997, openly
admitted 'I'd rather section nine people inappropriately and go O.T.T.
and take one dangerous person into hospital than have that dangerous
person on the streets'.

An inquiry culture has emerged which is worryingly reminiscent of
the child abuse scandals of the late 1980s (Franklin and Parton, 1991;
Parton, 1991). Mental health professionals, like their social work
counterparts in the child care field, have been subjected to a continual
bombardment of hastily prepared policies and guidelines. While it is
clearly right to question, and if necessary correct, bad practice, if this
is done in an atmosphere characteristic of a witch-hunt, then all that
will result is defensive practice and no progress will be made. For
Busfield (1996: 233) the key issue 'is not the absence or presence of
regulation, but on what grounds, for what purposes, and in whose
interests any regulation occurs'. She urges a move away from the
simplistic notion that 'care' and 'control' are mutually exclusive

strategies, arguing that both can only be reconciled once there is an explicit consideration of the values at stake in judgements concerning risk and dangerousness.

According to Muijen (1995: 44) 'the crisis in mental health care has much in common with other value-led issues society has to resolve. Mental health care is difficult to deliver perfectly, and seems to produce scandals and moral panics whichever way services are organized'. To this extent it would be naïve to suggest that the responsibility for the current moral panic should be laid exclusively at the door of the media. It has to be acknowledged that much of the recent public outrage and anxiety is rooted in long-standing and deep-rooted fears in society about madness and about psychiatry's ability to deal with it (Bott, 1975; Jodelet, 1991; Taylor, 1994/95). As Francis (1996: 4) notes, 'with the closure of the old psychiatric hospitals, the comfortable walls which separated madness from the "community" for 200 years are beginning to crumble'. Similarly, Prior observes:

> We have an acknowledged crisis in inner city mental health services, a serious retrenchment in social services provision and a loss of public confidence in the concept of community care.
>
> (1998: 22)

New Labour has pronounced that 'Care in the community has failed' (Frank Dobson, Health Secretary, House of Commons, 29 July 1998). Another review of the *Mental Health Act* is under way beneath the banner *Safe, Sound and Supportive* (Department of Health, 1998). While there are some positive noises about improving caring services for all those in mental distress, the overriding tone perpetuates the climate of fear of the mentally distressed:

> Care in the community has failed because, while it improved the treatment of many people who were mentally ill, it left far too many walking the streets, often at risk to themselves and a nuisance to others. We are going to ... ensure that patients who might otherwise be a danger to themselves and others are no longer allowed to refuse to comply with the treatment they need.
>
> (Frank Dobson cited in Department of Health, 1998)

Although the Government talks of its desire to meet the needs of the three primary 'stakeholders' in the field of mental distress – the patient, the carer(s) and the wider public – it is likely that the patients' 'needs' will continue to be defined by people other than themselves.

While the politicians and professionals prioritize their agendas around 'assertive outreach' and 'community treatment orders' allowing for the forcible treatment of patients in the community, by contrast, people with mental health problems define their needs in terms of far more ordinary things – affordable housing, access to employment, realistic benefit levels, a social life, help and support when in crisis, respect and trust, information and choice (Pilgrim, 1993; Prior, 1998).

As this century draws to a close, our society is demonstrating very little tolerance towards the mentally distressed. Attitudes are hardening and the value system of mental health care appears to be in disarray. There is a fundamental distrust in the legitimacy of psychiatric theory and practice epitomized in the headline 'We're mad to trust shrinks' (*Daily Mirror*, 9 February 1996: 7). Moreover, a national survey in 1995 reported that some 88 per cent of psychiatrists admitted to wanting to leave the profession (*Hospital Doctor*, 14 September 1995). In a BBC television programme reflecting on the history of the pioneering humanitarian spirit within psychiatry (*Pioneers*, 9 September 1996), one of the founders of the open-door movement, the psychiatrist David Clark quite tersely remarked that 'a society gets the psychiatry it deserves'. It remains to be seen whether psychiatry can sufficiently reinvent itself to be considered by both the public and service users to have a legitimate role in the provision of mental health care into the new millennium.

7 Towards a new critical perspective on mental health care

Beginning critical analysis

Since the Second World War there have been many developments in the theory and practice of mental health care. These include the emergence of various critiques of mainstream psychiatry, the proliferation of different schools of psychotherapy and a succession of challenges to psychiatric and psychotherapeutic orthodoxy. Additionally, in the British context, a succession of scandals in psychiatric hospitals during the 1970s (Martin, 1984) plunged the mental health services even deeper into a crisis of legitimacy which had begun to unfold with the publication of Russell Barton's *Institutional Neurosis* in 1959. Nevertheless, there has been no sustained effort to develop an integrated critical analysis of the theory and practice of mental health care which takes account of all these developments. Books by Lucy Johnstone (1989) and Parker *et al.* (1995) have gone some way towards developing such an analysis, while literature such as Phil Thomas's (1997) book about schizophrenia provides in-depth critical analysis of competing discourses of certain specific forms of mental distress. In this chapter we draw on the methodology of critical criminology in an attempt to take some tentative steps towards the development of an all-encompassing critical model of mental health, mental distress and psychotherapeutics. As there are already many competing perspectives on mental health it would be naïve to pretend that we are able to offer a definitive critical model of mental distress. Rather, we attempt to show how overlaps and tensions between various Western conceptions of mental health, mental distress and psychotherapeutic intervention might be subjected to systematic critical analysis.

One of the major constraints on the development of a critical approach is the existence of many different schools of psychotherapy:

The very fact that there are so many different schools of thought is worrying. One survey suggests there are over 450 schools of psychotherapy formally recognized in the West. There are probably a lot more actually, not so formally recognized. And we have to ask the question, "Why are there so many different schools of thought over the same problem?". And many of these schools have fundamentally opposing viewpoints. I mean, how can they co-exist?

(Persaud, 1995)

As the above quotation implies, there are major differences of opinion about what form psychotherapy should take. Thus it would be difficult to develop a meaningful analysis of so many competing perspectives within the constraints of any single book. Furthermore, this problem is compounded by a lack of empirical evidence that any form of psychotherapy is clinically effective (Stancombe and White, 1998). Therefore, as we explained in Chapter 3, we have confined our analysis of counselling and psychotherapy to those schools of psychotherapy which have had the greatest influence on clinical approaches to mental health care within the statutory mental health services.

In addition to the problems affecting critical analysis of psychotherapy, there is the problem that psychotherapy is only one approach to the understanding and management of mental distress and mental health. Medical psychiatry, clinical psychology and the various critical perspectives on mental health and mental distress must also be taken into consideration. Moreover, there are divisions within medical psychiatry and clinical psychology and the proponents of competing perspectives often seem to be more interested in promoting their own particular philosophies than learning from the work of those who do not share their perspectives. Consequently, humanistic insights and ground-breaking interventions developed by mental health professionals of previous generations are often overlooked by would-be radical practitioners.

A further problem is the broad spectrum of disorders covered by the American Psychiatric Association's current Diagnostic and Statistical Manual (APA, 1994) and the Mental Disorders section of the World Health Organization's current International Classification of Diseases (WHO, 1992). Although there is heated debate over the aetiology of some of the disorders, the aetiology of others listed is unambiguously biological (for example, some acute confusional states and degenerative conditions of the brain). While there are psychosocial interventions which may be helpful to those who suffer from such conditions, the critical approach which we propose is meant to apply only to those forms of mental distress for which there is no unambiguous evidence of biological or biochemical causation. These include psycho-neuroses, affective disorders, schizophreniform disorders, personality disorders and eating disorders such as bulimia and anorexia nervosa.

Some of these issues may be addressed by applying the method of enquiry associated with critical criminology to the study of mental health and mental distress. The key elements to critical criminological research are consideration of historical issues, ideological influences on 'common sense' assumptions, the socio-political contexts in which policy is developed and the impact which the interplay of these factors has on the experience of individuals. When this model is applied to the study of mental health, mental distress and mental health care, we are forced to ask certain questions. How did mental health services, which were inspired by the 'moral treatment' regime of the York Retreat in the late eighteenth century, deteriorate to the extent that human rights abuses were reported in some of Britain's psychiatric hospitals during the 1970s? How is it, that despite the emergence of anti-psychiatry in the 1960s, popular discourses of mental distress in the 1990s still suggest that 'schizophrenia' is inextricably linked to dangerousness? How and why do policy-makers uncritically accept certain theoretical perspectives on mental health and mental distress, while ignoring other competing perspectives? To what extent do political, social, cultural and economic factors contribute to the mental health or mental distress of individuals? What is the basis of institutionalized racism and sexism in mental health services and how can it be eradicated?

While the appropriateness of applying the theoretical approach of critical criminology to the study of mental health issues may be demonstrated by these questions, there are also important questions which such an approach does not address. In the context of mental health and mental distress there are two other factors which must also be considered. The first of these is socio-biology. Although it is not always clear whether biochemical changes are the cause of mental distress or the consequence of mental distress, there is evidence that biochemical changes are associated with certain forms of mental distress (Hedaya, 1996; Thomas, 1997). Even though biologically based research into schizophrenia continues to be inconclusive, the link between anxiety and activity of the autonomic nervous system is an indisputable biological fact, while the biological aspects of

Seasonal Affective Disorder (SAD) are widely acknowledged. For example, the fact that light therapy is an effective treatment for SAD is usually explained in biological terms.

The second additional factor which must be accounted for is the existence of competing *critiques* of psychiatry and psychotherapy. As there are valid points in each of these critiques and there is both overlap and tension between them (not least the tension between those that believe that psychotherapy is a useful intervention and those that believe that it is not), some analysis of these critiques should be incorporated into any discussion of ideology. Thus, although we have focused only on the most influential of the major schools of psychotherapy, our own critical approach to mental health and mental distress incorporates consideration of the relatively obscure psychiatric theories of the psychotherapist, Wilhelm Reich and the psychiatrist, Frantz Fanon. The rationale behind this is that there are elements in Fanonian and Reichian thought which resonate with and lend support to some of the later critiques of psychiatry. Furthermore, Fanon's work explicitly addresses the relationship between racism and mental distress.

While Fanon did not found an independent school of psychotherapy and neither Fanon nor Reich developed explicit critiques of psychiatry, both suggested that there is an interplay of socio-political and biological factors which contributes to the causation of mental distress. More importantly, both Reich and Fanon implicitly challenged the assumptions of mainstream psychiatry and psychotherapy and attempted to describe something akin to what Stancombe and White (1998) describe as 'post-therapeutics'. For example, Reich implies that the incidence of mental distress could be reduced through the eradication of authoritarianism and externally imposed moralism (Reich, 1975a, 1975b) while Fanon writes of the psychotherapeutic benefits of actively participating in resistance against oppression. Thus, Reich and Fanon both suggest practical alternatives to psychopharmacology and psychotherapy. Such ideas prefigure the work of the later anti-psychiatrists and should be considered alongside them.

The importance of history

As discussed in Chapter 1, theorists of mental health have often disregarded the complexities of history. For example, for many years textbooks of psychiatry implied that the history of psychiatry since the opening of the York Retreat in the 1790s has been one of uninterrupted progress and increasing humanitarianism. Notwithstanding the publication of Montagu Lomax's controversial *The Experiences of an Asylum Doctor* in 1921, this orthodoxy was rarely challenged until academics from other disciplines began to study the history of mental health services during the 1960s and 1970s. Since then, historians writing from both liberal and radical perspectives continue to offer a more balanced historical account. For example, Kathleen Jones writes of 'good intentions going wrong' (Jones, 1993: 3), while Andrew Scull offers a credible explanation for how and why the humanistic aspirations of 'moral treatment' became compromised as the asylum population mushroomed (Scull, 1993). The importance of the observations of these academics was underlined during the 1970s when a series of official inquiries discovered neglect, corruption and mistreatment in several large British psychiatric hospitals (Martin, 1984). Nevertheless, the brief historical notes in many textbooks of psychiatry tend to gloss over the historical failures and shortcomings of mental health services (for example, Anderson and Trethowan, 1973; Sim, 1981). Conversely, critics of psychiatry are wont to focus on abuses of psychiatry (for example, Survivors Speak Out, 1997) and ignore psychiatry's positive contributions. For example, notwith-standing the ethical and political debates about the legitimacy of forensic psychiatry, the psychiatric profession has been instrumental in establishing the legal principle that an offence may be partially mitigated if at the time of committing an offence, the accused did not know the nature and the quality of the act s/he was doing, or if s/he did know it, s/he did not know she was doing wrong (the McNaghten rule). Also, more fundamentally, medical psychiatrists have tradition-ally sought to lessen the stigma of mental distress by defining it as treatable illness. While this medicalization of mental distress has brought problems of its own, it absolved the distressed person from blame for his/her condition and challenged the view that mental distress was the consequence of moral degeneracy.

Curiously, a historical perspective is conspicuously lacking in the writings of R. D. Laing and others associated with the Philadelphia Association, although a historical perspective is an important dimension to the work of Thomas Szasz. While anti-psychiatry in general and the work of R. D. Laing in particular has stimulated many mental health professionals to think critically about their practice, the lack of a coherent historical perspective is problematic. Significantly, Laing failed to acknowledge the contributions which Carl Jung had made to the understanding of psychosis, the work of progressive medical superintendents of large psychiatric hospitals such as Bertram Mandelbrote and David Clark, or the development of a democratic

psychiatry by Tom Main, Maxwell Jones and other leading lights in
the therapeutic community movement (see Kennard, 1998). Inasmuch
as they all undertook work which in some sense prefigured the work of
Laing, this is somewhat surprising; not least because he was clearly
prepared to borrow ideas from other academic disciplines such as
philosophy. For someone who otherwise adopted an eclectic approach
to understanding mental distress, Laing's apparent failure to recognize
the importance of history was a curious oversight.

More recently, it is noticeable that advocates of psychological
treatments of schizophrenia (such as Marius Romme, John Watkins
and various cognitive therapists) have paid relatively little attention to
the contribution of the anti-psychiatrists to the development of
psychological treatments of psychosis (see Haddock and Slade, 1996;
Romme and Escher, 1993; Watkins, 1996). Examples of significant
contributions to the psychological management of psychosis by anti-
psychiatrists which have been overlooked in this literature include:
Morton Schatzman's (*circa* 1980) book *The Story of Ruth*, which
admittedly is not well known; Joseph Berke's oft-cited (1979) *I
Haven't Had to Go Mad Here* and R. D. Laing's (1965) classic work,
The Divided Self.

When the historical dimension is taken into account systematically,
it becomes apparent that there are (at least) two separate histories of
psychiatric thought and psychiatric care. These are the history of
general trends and the history of alternative approaches. However,
although both proponents of mainstream psychiatry and critics of
mainstream psychiatry tend to be selective when considering historical
perspectives, the boundaries between these two histories are not always
clear. For example, the work undertaken by physicians such as William
Battie and Thomas Withers in the early eighteenth century, as well as
the opening of the York Retreat in the 1790s, belong to both traditions. While the 'moral treatment' developed by these pioneers was
radical and innovative at the time, it was the model on which many
nineteenth century psychiatrists based their practice, albeit in a diluted
form (see Scull, 1993). Thus, although 'moral treatment' was in its time
a genuinely radical development, it is also the foundation on which the
psychiatric profession was built. In a slightly different context, the
work of The Tavistock Institute is widely respected in the worlds of
mainstream psychiatry, clinical psychology and psychotherapy, but is
also connected with the work of R. D. Laing inasmuch as Laing
undertook psychoanalytical training there and was working there
when his first books were published. Furthermore, during Laing's time
at the Tavistock Institute, he was instrumental in Tavistock Publica-

tions publishing the first ever English translation of Michel Foucault's *Madness and Civilisation* (Mullan, 1995); a book which subsequently influenced many English-speaking critics of psychiatry.

A further dimension to the overlap between the history of general trends and the history of alternative approaches is that certain alternative approaches might not have evolved but for changes taking place in mainstream psychiatry. For example, orthodox histories of psychiatry frequently suggest that it was the development of the phenothiazines and other new psychotropic drugs which made it possible to experiment more with using talking therapies with psychotic patients. While some writers suggest that the importance of these drugs to the transformation of psychiatric practice has been exaggerated, it is noteworthy that the use of other (high-risk) physical treatments, such as prefrontal leucotomy and insulin therapy, declined as the use of these drugs became widespread.

We have dealt with the history of general trends earlier in this book, so here we focus only on the history of what we have termed alternative approaches. These approaches are characterized by openness to new ideas about what causes mental distress and the development of innovative approaches to caring for people experiencing such distress. Although 'moral treatment' was the first such development, there seems to have been a period between the demise of moral treatment in the mid-nineteenth century and the beginning of the First World War, during which there were no major radical developments in social psychiatry and dynamic psychiatry. Then, during and after the First World War, mainstream medical psychiatry began to incorporate some ideas borrowed from psychoanalytical theory (Jones, 1993; Pilgrim and Rogers, 1993). This is significant because it paved the way for the birth of the therapeutic community movement at Northfield and Mill Hill military hospitals during the Second World War. Notwithstanding Laing and Cooper's failure to mention this work in any detail in their own writing, their work at (respectively) Kingsley Hall and Villa 21 is clearly located in this tradition (Kennard, 1998). Furthermore, the emergence of a credible mental health service users' movement during the 1980s owes some of its success to the part played by anti-psychiatry in challenging psychiatry's assumptions during the 1960s and 1970s. Therefore, the success of the service users' movement is indirectly linked to the history of the therapeutic community movement. Thus, it is possible to identify a tradition of democratic approaches to mental health care which began to emerge during the 1940s and has continued to exist on the margins of mainstream psychiatry ever since.

In order to gain a proper understanding of how our understanding of mental health, mental distress and mental health care has developed, this history of alternative approaches must be incorporated into the wider historical perspective. In order to do this effectively it is necessary to consider the issue of ideology.

The role of ideology

'Ideology' has been termed 'one of the most debated concepts in sociology' and it is a term which is used by different authors in different ways (Abercrombie *et al.*, 1988: 118). In the following discussion it refers to beliefs, assumptions and theories for which there is some circumstantial evidence but for which there is not yet incontrovertible evidence. As there is no undisputed scientific explanation of the origins of mental distress, all perspectives on mental health are ideologies in this sense.

As Stephen Pattison (1997) argues in his analysis of managerialism, such ideologies have more in common with theological creeds than with academic theories. Indeed, those who adopt such ideologies are wont to cling tenaciously to their chosen faith. Once a therapist has chosen to pledge allegiance to a particular theory, he or she will often accept uncritically the teachings of one particular theorist or group of theorists and even condemn any direct criticism of their chosen 'guru' or his/her teaching. Thus, mainstream medical psychiatry continues to treat Laing and Szasz as virtual heretics (for example, Kerr, 1997), while some admirers of Laing overlook his initially voluntary withdrawal from the NHS and his later professional misdemeanours and portray him as the victim of a vengeful medical establishment (Hinchliffe, 1991; Virden, 1996; cf. Laing, 1994). Similarly, many subscribers to Freudian theories of psychoanalysis are hostile to the revisionist perspectives developed by Melanie Klein and her followers (Kohon, 1986). A similar ideological bias is evident in the blinkered approach of many of those offering 'new' perspectives on mental health. For example, Fred Newman pays relatively little attention to the anti-psychiatry of Laing and Cooper (see Newman, 1991; Newman and Holzman, 1993a, 1993b) despite Laing and Cooper's links to the left-wing counter-culture of the 1960s and 1970s and Newman's professed Marxism. Similarly, few feminist theorists of mental health acknowledge the similarities between radical feminist critiques of patriarchal nuclear families and David Cooper's ideas about the role of families in contributing to mental distress (see Cooper, 1972).

The adoption of such narrow ideological perspectives on the part of theorists and practitioners of mental health has negative consequences. First, it leads to biased editorial policies in academic journals and biased curricula for mental health professional education programmes (Double, 1992; Thomas and Bracken, 1999). This, in turn, is reflected in the ideological narrow-mindedness of many practising psychiatrists (Roberts, 1990) and may also explain the arrogant self-promotion of some psychotherapists referred to by David Pilgrim (1997). Consequently, many mental health professionals are unaware of the extent of the difference of opinion as to what benefits mental health, what causes mental distress and how mental distress may be managed effectively. Therefore, many mental health professionals may genuinely believe that they offer a comprehensive range of treatment options to their clients when they are in fact only offering three or four out of dozens, if not hundreds, of possible interventions.

These problems are compounded by the way in which popular culture represents discourses of mental distress and psychotherapy as if they were scientific fact, rather than philosophical speculation. Thus, many members of the general public now have an unquestioning belief that people who have suffered certain kinds of emotional and psychological trauma have an objective need for counselling or psychotherapy (see Charlton, 1998). For example, in television and newspaper discussions of bereavement and disaster and, in television talk shows hosted by presenters such as Oprah Winfrey and Jerry Springer, such ideologies are never far beneath the surface. Notwithstanding the various critiques of psychiatric coercion, the power of the mental health professions at the turn of the twenty-first century would seem to be derived as much from popular faith in the validity of psychiatric and psychotherapeutic ideology as from legislation and social policy.

Such popular acceptance of psychiatric and/or psychotherapeutic ideology may pose problems for distressed individuals. Although many activists in the mental health service users' movement claim that no one can legitimately claim to have expertise in understanding another person's distress, distressed individuals may fear that their friends and associates will not view their situation sympathetically unless they seek professional help. In other words, even if psychosocial explanations of mental distress are accepted, distressed individuals are unlikely to get much sympathy unless they adopt the 'sick role' as elaborated by Talcott Parsons (1951), albeit seeking help from a counsellor or psychotherapist rather than a physician. (According to Parsons, illness is a form of deviance, but the sick person will be absolved of blame and exempted from social responsibilities as long as s/he seeks professional help from a physician and complies with any prescribed treatment regimen.) However, when professional help is sought, most mental health professionals will try to understand a client's distress by pursuing lines of enquiry which are predetermined by a particular theoretical perspective. Jeffrey Masson provides a good example of the pitfalls of this process in his discussion of the family therapist Ross Speck's observation that where a small child has sat in his/her father's favourite chair, this may indicate that a 'weak and passive father has abdicated his role in the family' (Masson, 1990: 250). Here the therapist interprets a mundane event as a sign of family dysfunction. Regrettably this is not an aberration: such fanciful interpretations are a common theme in psychoanalytical literature.

At the level of interaction between individual mental health professionals and individual service users, this is not necessarily problematic. For example, a client may be confident enough to challenge a therapist's incorrect interpretation of his/her actions, to change therapists, or to seek help from an alternative mental health service. However, there are also other implications. When it comes to formulating mental health policy, certain theoretical perspectives are more appealing to politicians than others. For example, politicians (whatever their political persuasion) are less likely to be comfortable with a perspective that links mental distress to economic depression and political repression than with a perspective that emphasizes the genetic factors which contribute to the causation of mental distress. Similarly, politicians may prefer to support low-cost and relatively poor-quality mental health services rather than relatively high-cost, highest quality mental health services which could only be funded through massive increases in taxation. Indeed, the myth that community care has 'failed' and that more secure provision is required for mentally distressed individuals is, at least partly, a reflection of such considerations (Perkins, 1999a; Taylor and Gunn, 1999). Specifically, there has been a lack of political will to significantly increase the level of funding of mental health services as psychiatric hospitals have closed down and services have been moved into the community.

The importance of social and political structures

One of the dominant themes in the direct critiques of mental health services associated with writers such as Szasz, Laing, Cooper, Scull and Foucault is the contention that mental health services (especially those which are funded by the state) have an important social control function. Inasmuch as this claim is made by writers who approach the issue from a variety of political perspectives, it would seem reasonable to assume that there is some validity to this point of view. Additionally, it is a view which is supported by anti-racist and feminist writers who point to psychiatry's links with eugenics, neo-colonialism and patriarchy. However, the social control function of British psychiatry has never been overt in the way that it was in the former Soviet Union (see Cohen, 1989). Indeed, the political outcry which followed the conviction of Michael Stone for the murders of mother and daughter Lin and Megan Russell in 1998 suggests that psychiatry is ineffective as a technology of social control. Prior to Stone being charged with this offence, psychiatrists had refused to admit him to hospital on the grounds that he had an untreatable personality disorder. Following Stone's trial, some politicians criticized contemporary mental health policy and practice for failing to protect the public from dangerous individuals and proposed far-reaching changes to mental health law.

On the other hand, the political reaction to the case of Michael Stone apparently being refused psychiatric treatment on the grounds that he was not suffering from a treatable mental illness (Pilgrim 1999) does imply that politicians *expect* psychiatry to have a social control function. Furthermore, the widely reported incarceration of unmarried mothers in psychiatric hospitals in the earlier part of the twentieth century provides evidence that psychiatry has, at least historically, played a role in regulating social values and standards of behaviour and disciplining those who transgress.

Historical, ideological and socio-political factors come together to shape conceptions of mental health and responses to mental distress. For example, the historical dominance of the medical model of 'mental illness' underpins the popular conception of mentally distressed individuals as irrational and dependent upon the intervention of others. Although alternative discourses of mental distress are recognized and understood by some mental health professionals and mental health service users, it is clearly this popular conception of mental distress which is behind policy initiatives such as supervision registers and legislative measures such as compulsory treatment orders and supervised discharge orders.

Another dimension to the relationship between history, ideology and politics and conceptions of mental distress is evident in the relationship between psychiatry, eugenics and Nazi euthanasia policies. As Suman Fernando (1991) argues, the emergence of psychiatry as a distinct medical discipline in the nineteenth century coincided with the emergence of eugenics and Darwinian theory. During the 1930s, Nazi psychiatrists in Hitler's Germany defended their policy of 'euthanasia' of learning disabled and chronically mentally ill individuals by appealing to eugenic theory (Breggin, 1973; Burleigh, 1994). Although it may be argued that the Nazi psychiatrists behaved in this way because they were Nazis, rather than because they were psychiatrists, this highlights the problem of the relationship between psychiatry and eugenics, and raises the question of why the professional ethics of psychiatry did not deter them from acting in this way. An appreciation of these issues is crucial to understanding why many users of mental health services are suspicious of research into the biological causes of mental distress. While it is difficult to imagine any psychiatrist today seriously proposing a euthanasia policy, nascent medical technologies such as gene therapy combined with acceptance of the principle of compulsory treatment herald the possibility of highly invasive treatments being inflicted upon mentally distressed persons against their will.

While most biological psychiatrists and academic socio-biologists are sensitive to these issues and understand the complex nature of the relationship between environmental and genetic factors, these fears are understandable. Since the late nineteenth century, mental health law has given psychiatrists incredible direct power over those referred to them. Furthermore, mental health services are organized in such a way that other mental health professionals may be able to influence psychiatrists and thereby indirectly exert similar power over service users. Although most mental health professionals use this power in ways which they genuinely believe are in service users' best interests, mistakes are easily made. Indeed, there is a long history in psychiatry of aggressive application of physical interventions which are later shown to be of questionable value. These include prefrontal leucotomy, insulin therapy, electro-convulsive therapy and long-term prescription of minor tranquillizers such as diazepam (Valium) and chlordiazepoxide (Librium). Furthermore, there is evidence that, despite checks and balances being built into the system, individual mental health professionals may behave in an oppressive manner towards those in their care (Blom-Cooper, 1992; Martin, 1984). Thus, suspicions about biological research into mental distress and how such research might be used cannot be dismissed as mere paranoia.

The biological dimension in perspective

The influence which Darwinism and eugenics has had on the development of psychiatry is reflected in the attitude of those psychiatrists who have unquestioning faith in the methodology of the natural sciences and reject discourses of mental distress which arise from other perspectives. Although there may be relatively few psychiatrists with such blinkered vision, Phil Thomas (1997) suggests that such a faction still exists within the Royal College of Psychiatrists. In contrast to the apparent belief in biological determinism on the part of some psychiatrists, modern socio-biologists tend to believe that human behaviour is shaped by a complex interplay of genetic and environmental factors (Ridley, 1993). Similarly, progressive biological psychiatrists recommend multi-modal therapeutic responses to mental distress rather than purely physical interventions (Farmer and Owen, 1996; Hedaya, 1996; Watkins, 1996). Admittedly such theorists tend to place greater emphasis on biological factors than on anything else. However, the fact that they consider other factors to be relevant opens up the possibility of meaningful dialogue between mental health professionals who subscribe to such theories and mental health service users who are sceptical of the value of biological research into mental distress.

Unfortunately, though, many writers argue that there is something inherently immoral about discussing whether or not there is a biological dimension to mental distress. Thomas Szasz is of course the best known of these self-styled radicals but many service user activists share his concerns. The following quotations are typical of opinions on biological research expressed in literature written by service user activists:

> Today we root schizophrenia in all sorts of things. Some people root it in the family; some people root it in your biology. Some people root it in your genes. It is all nonsense. If you want to root schizophrenia in anything, root it in society because society needs schizophrenia.
>
> (Coleman, 1996/1997: 11)

> [Survivors Speak Out] call upon all survivors of [the] mental health system and their relatives to have nothing whatsoever to do with genetic testing in relation to mental disorder, either as part of research or as predictive tests.
>
> (Roberts, 1997: 10)

The articles from which these passages are taken contain valid criticisms of psychiatric coercion, and the historical link between eugenics and Nazi psychiatry certainly renders their views understandable. Nevertheless, they are antithetical to the principles of developing an authentically critical perspective on mental health because the authors of these articles refuse to accept the legitimacy of certain kinds of research. The flaw in this kind of thinking may be demonstrated with reference to the question of medication.

The accusation that many psychiatrists over-emphasize the role of medication in the management of mental distress is a valid one. However, there is no logical inconsistency in believing that one's mental distress has been precipitated by socio-political factors and taking medication to control one's natural and/or learnt responses to those events. In principle, this is no different to taking paracetamol to ease the pain of a headache caused by stress or overtiredness. The problem arises when the belief that one's distress has been provoked by socio-political circumstances is denied, ridiculed or invalidated (Fanon, 1967) and/or a person is coerced into taking medication against their will. The critics quoted above do not remove the problem of positivist medical psychiatry, but merely invert it by substituting one orthodoxy for another.

If a person freely chooses to manage his/her distress through taking medication, why should s/he be prevented from doing so? If a person does wish to take medication, the chosen solution is far more likely to be effective if s/he takes medication which has been specifically designed to control those symptoms. Research into the correlation between particular forms of mental distress and particular human biochemistry would increase the likelihood that truly effective psychotropic medications with less side effects will eventually be developed (see Hedaya, 1996). In this sense, the importance of biological research into mental distress is clear. On the other hand, there is a need to protect users of mental health services from being coerced into accepting interventions which may be of little value to them, particularly if those interventions have unpleasant side effects.

Mental distress as human experience

While it is important not to ignore socio-biology, its contributions to our understanding of human experience and human behaviour must be put into perspective. In particular, it is important not to fall into the trap of obsessive postivism and dismiss as invalid anything which cannot be indisputably proven to be true. The problem of this approach can be demonstrated by considering the question of the existence of God. God's existence cannot be proven but, notwithstanding the existence of religious wars and the occasional persecution of individuals by dogmatic and insensitive clergy, millions of people testify that their faith in God has given them strength and courage.

Indeed, some people claim that their religious faith has helped them cope with mental distress, while others claim they have received a vocation from God to care for mentally distressed individuals. Thus, whatever one's personal beliefs and feelings on the subject, it would be ridiculous to dismiss the concept of God as being irrelevant to human experience.

To return to the question of mental distress, there is a long history of people having experiences which psychiatrists would regard as 'psychotic' and coping with them. There are examples in the Old Testament for instance, such as the 'hallucinations' and what might have been a catatonic stupor described by the prophet Ezekiel (Ezekiel, 1: 1–28 and 3: 25 to 4: 1–8, respectively). During the late nineteenth century psychic researchers collected apparently reliable data about visual hallucinations, telepathy (cf. passivity feelings and thought insertion in psychiatric parlance) and out-of-body experiences (cf. de-realization and depersonalization in psychiatric parlance) in subjects who had no psychiatric history (Broad, 1962). However, it would be naïve to romanticize all such experiences. For many people, such experiences are truly terrifying, even if they are able to bring them under their conscious control (see Romme and Escher, 1993; Schatzman, *circa* 1980). Furthermore, not all mental distress is 'exotic'. While it is possible to retrospectively ascribe hidden meanings to psychotic symptoms and redefine them as spiritual enlightenment or Maslowian peak experiences, it is more difficult to think of uncontrollable anger, acute panic attacks, deep depression or attempted suicide in a positive way.

On the other hand, the fact that people who do not have psychiatric histories sometimes hallucinate suggests that such phenomena may be within the range of normal human experiences. Also, evidence that some people can learn to manage their hallucinations suggests that physical treatments are not the only way of controlling the distress caused by such experiences, and may not necessarily be the most effective response. It is also worthy of note that this is not altogether a recent discovery. During the twentieth century, the idea that even psychotic forms of mental distress may be meaningful to the person experiencing them and can sometimes be understood by others occurs in several schools of psychotherapeutic thought.

Carl Gustav Jung suggested that 'psychosis' was a particularly severe form of mental distress which was further along the same continuum as 'neurosis' (Jung, 1977) and, like Laing, believed that the apparently 'meaningless' content of psychotic ideas could be understood (Jung, 1961). Indeed, in his autobiography, he describes personal inner experiences which may at least partly explain how he came to these conclusions. These include visions which he had during the first half of 1914 and how these seemed to represent a connection between his own personal crises at that time and the events which ultimately led to the outbreak of the First World War (Jung, 1961: 199f). Additionally, although he was somewhat pessimistic about the value of psychotherapy as a treatment for psychosis, he suggests that early treatment with psychotherapy might prevent the onset of psychotic symptoms (Jung, 1977). Thus, Jung's views on psychosis seem to imply that he believed psychotic experience to be something which, depending on external circumstances, might affect any human being.

Although Jung, Romme, the so-called anti-psychiatrists and cognitive therapists have gone furthest in suggesting how psychotic experiences may be understood and worked with psychotherapeutically, they are not alone in expounding this viewpoint. For example, Eric Berne, founder of Transactional Analysis, suggests psychosocial explanations for how individuals might develop schizophrenia or affective disorders (Berne, 1975). Similarly, at least one Gestalt therapist claims partial success in treating a person with a diagnosis of chronic schizophrenia (Van Dusen, 1975).

Nevertheless, whatever the merits of these perspectives on mental distress, the medicalization of mental distress persists. Certainly, there is widespread acceptance of the validity of alternative approaches such as counselling and psychotherapy to manage the stresses of everyday life and neurotic conditions such as free-floating anxiety, reactive depression and phobias. However, when it comes to 'personality disorders' and psychoses (especially schizophrenia), the public debate about mental health policy is still dominated by medical discourses of mental disorder. Thus, in debates about mental health policy, those who are considered to have such problems are almost invariably discussed in terms of being irrational, potentially dangerous and needing to be monitored and controlled as well as cared for (Crepaz-Keay, 1998; Department of Health, 1998; Pedler and Foster 1998; Pilgrim, 1999). On the other hand, another dimension to these same debates about mental health policy is the notion of 'working in partnership'.

Resistance or partnership?

Where 'working in partnership' refers to inter-agency working (for example, health services, social services and housing services working in partnership) this concept is unproblematic. On the other hand, Thomas (1997) suggests that it is fundamentally dishonest to refer to partnership between service users and professionals, because of the power difference between them. Such power difference is particularly important in respect of Approved Social Workers (under the 1983 *Mental Health Act*), GPs and psychiatrists who, together, have the power to compulsorily detain mentally distressed persons who will not agree to treatment. However, there are also more subtle ways in which the power of mental health professionals is significant. For example, where psychiatrists (or other mental health professionals) who do not fully understand the relevant issues, find themselves in the role of gatekeepers to other services. This is often the case with people with transsexual syndrome or gender dysphoria, who may in the first instance be referred to psychiatric services by their GPs rather than to gender identity clinics. This may result in unnecessary delays in gaining access to appropriate professional help as the training of mental health professionals tends to focus on common mental health problems rather than on the more obscure conditions which are listed in psychiatric diagnostic manuals (Redding, 1996). Consequently, few mental health professionals fully understand the predicament of gender dysphoric or transsexual individuals and may therefore misinterpret their situation and delay referral to more appropriate specialist services.

Such power differentials have led Thomas (1997) to suggest that we should refer to 'alliances' rather than 'partnerships' between professionals and service users. It is clear from Thomas's own writing that he is committed to the development of democratic approaches to psychiatry. However, there are those who believe that the relationship between a psychiatrist (or other mental health professional) and a service user is inherently disempowering and that such alliances are therefore hopelessly idealistic. According to this viewpoint, the relationship between a mental health professional is a political struggle in which the service user is engaged in resisting oppressive interventions which the professional is attempting to impose upon him or her. This perspective is particularly evident in David Cooper's later books, the philosophy of the Campaign Against Psychiatric Oppression (CAPO) and, to some extent, in anti-racist perspectives on psychiatry (see Sashidharan, 1994).

To put these criticisms into perspective, the notion of therapeutic alliance is a recurring theme in the treatment and care of mentally distressed individuals. For example, notwithstanding Scull's assertion that the moral treatment of the eighteenth century was not liberal by twentieth century standards (Scull, 1993), it nevertheless emphasized the importance of not using coercion or restraint and appealing to the rationality of 'patients' to whatever extent that was possible. Some degree of therapeutic alliance is also necessary in any 'confessional' form of psychotherapy such as psychoanalysis and person-centred counselling, as well as in cognitive therapy. The most highly developed forms of therapeutic alliance are to be found in therapeutic community settings (with the possible exception of hierarchical 'concept houses' for people with addictions) (Kennard, 1998), and in social psychiatry (see Romme and Escher, 1993). However, therapeutic communities represent a very specialized form of mental health care, and there remains a need to develop strong conceptual frameworks for the practice of democratic psychiatry in wider contexts.

From critical theories to radical practice

It is relatively easy to identify and distinguish between historical, ideological and structural influences on the development of mental health services and the impact they have had on users of mental health services. However, translating such critical analysis into a conceptual model of democratic mental health care is a much more complex task. One way of doing this would be to use each successive critique of psychiatric orthodoxy to examine what has preceded it, but the overlap between the history of general trends in mental health care and the history of alternative approaches makes it difficult to identify an appropriate starting point. Also, while it is relatively easy to identify and analyse interactions between social and political structure and individual agency (i.e. the consequences of interaction between individual users of mental health services and individual mental health professionals), it is not always so easy to determine the practical implication of historical and ideological influences. Nevertheless, consideration of historical and ideological perspectives helps in clarifying what assumptions should underpin any critical perspective on mental health, mental distress and mental health care. For example, it is clear from the history of British mental health services that, at various times during the last two hundred years, both medical and psychosocial interventions have been successfully employed in the management of most forms of mental distress. Similarly, most radical psychiatrists (with the possible exception of Thomas Szasz) have been prepared to accept that there is some kind of legitimate role for the medical profession in the diagnosis and management of mental distress. For example, there is some evidence that David Cooper was not averse to the prescription of drugs (Conran, 1997; Sigal, 1986), while R. D. Laing believed that it was important to 'build a bridge between neurology and individual experience' (Mullan, 1995: 251). Likewise, neither Reich nor Fanon (both of whom suggested that political repression could precipitate mental distress) discounted the importance of considering the physiological dimension to mental distress. Furthermore, it is well known that it can be difficult to distinguish between certain forms of mental distress and certain endocrine, neurological, nutritional, infectious disorders or tumours. For these reasons – not to mention contemporary criticisms of other branches of Western allopathic medicine for failing to develop a holistic perspective – it is difficult to see a valid argument against the involvement of the medical profession in the diagnosis and management of mental distress or of research into biological dimensions to mental distress.

What does give cause for concern, however, is the subtle operation of a hierarchy of ideologies which seems to privilege discourses which incorporate biological psychiatry over all competing discourses. The 1983 *Mental Health Act* reflects this by giving power and authority to medical psychiatrists which is not granted to other mental health professionals. Within psychiatry, biologically biased psychiatrists seem to be more influential within medical psychiatry than social psychiatrists or those of an eclectic orientation. This is evident, for example, in the content of standard textbooks on psychiatry; in some of the policies formulated by the Royal College of Psychiatrists; in the differential allocation of research funding; and in the emphasis on the prescription of psychotropic medication which is characteristic of contemporary psychiatry (Healy *et al.*, 1998; Pilgrim and Rogers, 1993; Thomas and Bracken, 1999). While this hierarchy of theoretical perspectives exists *within* psychiatry, the legal status enjoyed by medically trained psychiatrists effectively renders all other psychological and psychotherapeutic perspectives less influential than any form of medical psychiatry (including those of psychiatrists, such as Joe Berke and the late R. D. Laing, who chose to practise mental health care outside the medical establishment). Those therapeutic approaches, such as cognitive therapy, which have been widely adopted by clinical psychologists (with their post-graduate professional education and relatively high professional status) are also held in high regard by policy-makers and politicians. However, other perspectives (such as counselling psychology) are less influential, despite having a populist appeal.

Although there is a sustained rhetoric on the part of the Government about 'working in partnership' and building a 'stakeholder society', it is difficult to determine where the perspectives of service users are located in this notional hierarchy of ideologies (Clarke and Newman, 1997; Pilgrim and Rogers, 1998). However, the mental health policies of recent Conservative governments and the current Labour government have put a lot of emphasis on surveillance of mentally distressed individuals and discretionary powers of psychiatrists to impose compulsory supervision and treatment orders on them (Crepaz-Keay, 1998; Thomas and Bracken, 1999). This would seem to imply that policy-makers are sceptical about the claims of the more radical factions within the users' movement that most mental distress can be managed effectively without the uninvited intervention of mental health professionals.

Anyone seriously committed to developing a critical model of mental health and mental distress needs to find ways of challenging this hierarchy of ideologies. Members of the medical profession have been involved in the care of mentally distressed persons for over two hundred years, and despite intensive research no unambiguous biological causative factors have been identified for any so-called mental disorders except the dementias and some acute confusional states. On the other hand, psychotropic drugs are useful in the management of mental distress in some individuals and it may not be a coincidence that the incidence of catatonic states has declined greatly since the introduction of the phenothiazine group of drugs in the 1950s (Jenner, 1996/1997). Numerous psychological and psychosocial theories of mental distress have also been formulated and many interventions based on these theories have been found to be effective with some individuals. However, few people who have been confronted by individuals in severe acute psychotic states would disagree that being with and communicating with such individuals may be difficult, frustrating, emotionally exhausting and sometimes even frightening. Indeed, Peter Sedgwick (1982) argued that Laing was only able to claim success in treating people at Kingsley Hall because he was not working with the most severely distressed individuals. On the other hand, there is now quite a lot of anecdotal and empirical evidence which shows that many psychotic symptoms can (at least sometimes) be managed successfully without resorting to medication (for example, Haddock and Slade, 1996; Romme and Escher, 1993).

On the basis of the foregoing discussion, it would seem that an authentically critical perspective on mental health and mental distress would need to be a bio-psychosocial one. Starting from the premise that there is nothing inherently wrong with the involvement of the medical profession in the diagnosis and management of mental distress, it is not difficult to develop a bio-psychosocial model of mental health and mental distress by applying various critiques to medical psychiatry. However, it is a much greater challenge to develop such a model of care which would also facilitate the development of effective therapeutic alliances between service users and mental health professionals. Part of the problem is that so-called theories of mental health are inconclusive. While sound theoretical arguments and/or empirical evidence can be cited in support of such theories, there are usually equally sound theoretical arguments and/or examples from practice which seemingly contradict them. Furthermore, some theories about mental health (such as those associated with Laing and Cooper, for example) reflect transitory intellectual trends, whereas others have more enduring appeal. Thus, on the one hand, medically orientated psychiatry (with its roots in empirical science) has remained relatively strong because of widespread respect for other scientific endeavour such as aviation, space travel, information technology and transplant surgery. On the other hand, alternative perspectives on mental health have tended to reflect relatively short-lived intellectual fashions and so have not been shaped into a coherent alternative perspective to med-ical psychiatry. Instead, psychoanalysis, behaviourism, therapeutic communities, Transactional Analysis, and person-centred counselling have all at some time or another captured the imagination of the intelligentsia, but interest has faded as social, political and intellectual trends have moved on. In addition to hindering the development of a coherent alternative to medical psychiatry, this has led to some useful therapeutic interventions passing into relative obscurity, only to be 'rediscovered' by subsequent generations of mental health profession-als and mental health service users. This lack of continuity is discernible, for example, in the history of British psychiatric nursing.

The 1968 Review of Psychiatric Nursing (Ministry of Health, 1968) identified best practice in psychiatric nursing, much of it based on the therapeutic community approach and group therapy. However, during the 1970s collectivism became unfashionable, so instead of building the 1983 syllabus of training for Registered Mental Nurses on the firm foundations identified in the 1968 Review, its authors proposed a radical new approach based on the then fashionable (and individualistic) Rogerian person-centred psychotherapy. This was problematic for two reasons. First, there is no evidence that Rogerian therapy is suitable for working with people with psychotic disorders and other chronic problems. Second, there were few people with expertise in Rogerian therapy in the mental health nursing profession at that time, so it was a very watered down model of Rogerian therapy which came to dominate the mental health profession (Hopton, 1997a; Hopton and Glenister, 1996). Consequently, it is now commonplace to meet mental health nurses who speak about showing 'unconditional positive regard' to service users but who are unable to articulate how exactly this might be demonstrated in a relationship with someone, or explain how such an approach might help someone suffering from severe psychosis.

Towards a new paradigm of mental health care

A truly anti-oppressive, anti-discriminatory model of mental health care should have the following characteristics. First, it should incorporate biological, psychological and social perspectives so that whatever the views of any service user there is a starting point for a dialogue between service user and professional which has the potential to develop into a therapeutic alliance. Second, inasmuch as all theories of mental health and mental distress are inconclusive, it should incorporate an explicit challenge to the notion that either psychological, social or biological perspectives are more important than the other two. Otherwise, potentially useful interventions might be overlooked. Third, it should have strong historical roots so that good practices are not swept away by the vagaries of fashion. Fourth, as contemporary psychiatric practice can be shown to result in race and sex discrimination, it should have an explicit anti-racist and anti-sexist dimension to it.

As indicated previously, it is difficult to pinpoint the most appropriate era in which such a model should be historically rooted. Nevertheless, the 1950s would seem to be a suitable place to start. This was the decade in which the use of physical treatments such as insulin therapy, electro-convulsive therapy and even psychosurgery was still commonplace; the therapeutic community movement was still growing; a significant minority of psychiatrists were interested in furthering their knowledge of psychoanalysis; and community-based psychiatry and new psychotropic drugs were being developed. Thus, although psychiatry in the 1950s was still bio-medically orientated, it had incorporated some psychological and social perspectives on mental health and mental distress. Furthermore, it is this relatively liberal psychiatry which was the target of the emerging critiques of psychiatry developed by sociologists such as Erving Goffman and Thomas Scheff and dissident psychiatrists such as Laing, Szasz and

Cooper as well as those developed later by feminist and anti-racist commentators. In developing their critiques of psychiatry, Szasz, Laing and the other anti-psychiatrists were trying to precipitate a move away from hospital-based psychiatry and bio-medical perspectives on mental health and mental distress. Although there are profound differences between the perspectives of Laing and Szasz, and even between those of Laing and Cooper, they share a distaste for compulsory detention and treatment of mentally distressed individuals which is echoed in the work of later critics of psychiatry such as Jeffrey Masson. At first, this critique of psychiatric coercion seems difficult to argue with. The charge that psychiatry is coercive is based on the assumption that acting against the will of even a severely distressed person is a violation of that person's basic human rights. However, even if it is accepted that a person's disturbing psychotic behaviour or self-harm has meaning, there may be sound ethical arguments for restraining people whose actions appear to be irrational (see Hopton, 1995). Therefore, a truly anti-oppressive model of mental health care must allow for the possibility that there will be times when it is justifiable to act against the will of a distressed person. Otherwise, would-be suicides who could not be persuaded to consider alternative courses of action would be left to die, while some severely delusional individuals might not get any kind of 'care' until they had lost their liberty for committing a criminal act. Indeed, it was precisely such a naïve interpretation of anti-oppressive mental health care which contributed to the chain of events which culminated in the killing of Jonathan Zito by Christopher Clunis (Ritchie *et al.*, 1994).

However, the observations of Laing, Cooper and Szasz, together with the evidence of many official inquiries into mental health care (Sheppard, 1996), leave us in no doubt that the rights of mental health service users can be and have been severely abused by negligent, untrustworthy or malicious mental health professionals. Moreover, the legal safeguards of service users' rights which have been incorporated into mental health legislation have often been ineffective (Coleman, 1996/1997; Walton 1996/1997). Thus, demands for self-determination and independent advocacy from activists within the mental health service users' movement are justified. However, there is clearly a need for a creative solution to the problem arising from the tension between these demands and the need to protect severely distressed individuals such as Christopher Clunis and Michael Stone from themselves and the public from them. There are no easy answers but, at the very least, there has to be transparency in procedures for assessing 'dangerousness' and recognition that the process of making such judgements is not and never can be an exact science. Human emotions and human behaviour are too complex for that ever to be a realistic expectation.

Furthermore, Szasz and the anti-psychiatrists showed that, whatever the biological dimension to mental distress might be, there are also psychosocial and socio-political dimensions to mental health and mental distress. This theme is also found in the work of earlier writers such as Fanon, Reich and members of the Frankfurt School of social scientists whose work incorporated the idea that personal and political issues are inseparable from each other (Fromm, 1979, 1990; Jay 1973). Additionally, it is implicit in the writings of the concentration camp survivor therapists, Heimler, Frankl and Bettelheim. However, it was Szasz and the anti-psychiatrists who developed the first explicit arguments that psychotherapeutic interventions, which assumed individual pathology, were problematic. More recently, socio-biologists have argued that the interaction between biological and environmental factors is extremely complex. Thus, 'dangerousness' is not a fixed and unchangeable condition but the product of particular political, social and environmental circumstances.

If mental health services are to be truly user-centred, certain factors must be taken into consideration. As there is evidence in support of biological, social and psychogenic factors being causative factors in the development of mental distress, care should be based on a bio-psychosocial model of aetiology and intervention. This would open up the possibility of dialogue, negotiation and compromise where mental health professionals and mental health service users have different opinions about the cause of mental distress. The development of such a user-centred service might encourage distressed persons who are sceptical about the value of medical models of mental illness/distress to utilize rather than avoid services. However, it would be naïve to assume that all mentally distressed persons – including those at risk of self-harm, self-neglect, harm to others or exploitation by others – would refer themselves to such services. The recent history of mental health services shows that there is a need for legal mechanisms to intervene in such circumstances, but that mental health professionals can be oppressively interventionist. Thus, there is a need for reliable and informed independent advocacy services, and mental health professionals to be honest enough to admit that their risk assessments are based as much on intuition and hunches as on reliable scientific theory. In a mental health service based on these principles it should be possible for service users and mental health professionals to develop truly egalitarian and democratic therapeutic alliances, wherein care and treatment are the product of honest negotiation rather than the expression of professional power. While this would address the conflict between the principle of freedom from coercion on the one hand, and the need to guarantee public safety and protect vulnerable individuals on the other, it does not address all critiques of mainstream mental health theories and mental health services. Any service will inevitably reflect the values and ideologies that are prevalent in the society where it is located. Thus, as long as class, race and sex prejudice are endemic in a society, they cannot be completely eradicated from a particular service which is provided within that society. Certainly, the effects of such prejudice and discrimination can be countered by making negotiation of care an absolute right and ensuring that appropriate advocacy services are properly funded. However, these measures do not address the problem that discrimination and prejudice may be significant factors in causing mental distress.

This leads to the socio-political understanding of mental distress associated with writers such as Reich, Fanon, Cooper and Newman. For each of these writers, oppression is a key factor in the causation of mental distress. Consequently, Reich and Fanon rejected conventional psychotherapy which focuses on 'insight' in favour of action which reaffirms one's sense of identity and self-worth. While Cooper and Newman are less concerned with questions of identity and self-esteem, they share with Fanon and, to a certain extent, Reich, a belief that collective political action is more useful than individual therapy. In this sense, their ideas prefigure Masson's plea for a moratorium on psychotherapy. However, Reich developed therapeutic interventions based on holism and political sociology, while Newman developed a therapy based on the principles of co-operativism and Vygotskian psychology. When these factors are considered alongside the apparent successes of the therapeutic community movement, the achievements of the mental health service users' movement and various pleas for the development of 'post-therapeutics', they seem to suggest that mental health care should be based on principles of collectivism, community development, and the active involvement of mental health professionals in political struggles against discrimination and oppression. Some of the difficulties of translating these principles into practice are considered in the final chapter.

8   Implications for practice

There are already many theories of causation of mental distress and it is difficult to see how any additional theoretical perspective could truly add anything to our understanding of mental distress, mental health or mental health care. Indeed, one of the most striking features of the history of mental health care is the way in which various writers, who claim to have developed new therapeutic interventions, seem to have in fact rediscovered older perspectives which have either fallen into relative obscurity as intellectual fashions have changed or have always been relatively unknown. For example, the milieu therapy and social therapy advocated by some psychiatrists during the 1950s and 1960s bears some resemblance to the ideals (if not the reality) of eighteenth and nineteenth century 'moral treatment'. Similarly, the ethos of Fred Newman's East Side Institute for Short-Term Psychotherapy has some resonance with the philosophies of some of the less psychoanalytically orientated therapeutic communities (see Kennard, 1998). To misquote a catchphrase from a cult television programme, the truth is already out there. The challenge for mental health professionals is to get beyond dogmatic adherence to any one particular theory on the one hand, and haphazard eclecticism on the other, so that they might discover it. In the previous chapter we suggested a framework of theoretical guidelines which may be applied to any combination of theories to aid constructive critical consideration of issues pertinent to mental health, mental distress and mental health care. In this final chapter, we set out the implications which we believe such a theoretical approach has for practice.

Professionals need to have some understanding of the history of mental health services and ideas about mental health. This is necessary for a number of reasons. First, this history is characterized by frequent changes in ideas about what kinds of therapy are of value in the management of mental distress. Thus, mental health professionals who do not have a historical perspective are prone to 'reinvent the wheel' when they devise experimental approaches to mental health care, and may overlook important developments by earlier practitioners. Second, quasi political challenges to dominant ideologies of mental health (such as those arising from the so-called anti-psychiatry of the 1960s and 1970s) are likely to be dismissed as aberrations and fads unless practitioners are aware of earlier politically orientated psychiatry such as the work of Reich or Fanon's psychosocial analysis of colonialism. Third, awareness that potentially useful therapeutic approaches may fade into obscurity as social, political and intellectual fashions change should discourage practitioners from uncritically assuming that less well-known therapeutic approaches such as Eugene Heimler's theory of Human Social Functioning are no longer of any relevance (see Heimler, 1967).

The case of medical psychiatry may be used to illustrate the importance of practitioners of mental health care being aware of how social, political and intellectual trends have affected ideologies of mental health. Medical psychiatry achieved its pre-eminent position among theories of mental health and mental distress at a time when patriarchy, imperialism, Darwinism and eugenics were in ascendancy. Consequently, sexism, racism and pessimism about the prognosis of mental distress may have become institutionalized into medical psychiatry at an early stage in its development. Mental health professionals who are aware of these connections are in a position to evaluate critically any theoretical perspectives which suggest that there are differences in the forms of mental distress experienced by men and women or people from different ethnic groups. Similarly, awareness of the close connection between anti-psychiatry and the counter-culture of the 1960s and 1970s enables professionals to distinguish between those pronouncements of Cooper and Laing which are merely reflections of the *zeitgeist* of that era, and those which are tacitly supported by other theoretical perspectives on mental health. Thus, the historically aware mental health professional is able to take account of the social and political dimensions to various perspectives on mental health and mental distress.

A historical perspective also enables mental health professionals to understand the implications of contemporary policy debates. The last generation of mental health professionals to have first-hand experience of working in overcrowded anti-therapeutic Victorian asylums are now in their forties. Thus, relatively few of today's mental health professionals have first-hand experience of the problems associated with the provision of long-term residential mental health care or of some of the more innovative ways in which these problems might be overcome. Many of the politicians, civil servants and health service administrators who now advocate reversing the policy of community care and developing more residential care for mentally distressed individuals are their contemporaries. In the absence of first-hand experience of mental health services based largely on residential care, these people may not appreciate the unique complexities associated with providing good quality user-centred residential care in the context of large organizations. Therefore, an understanding of the historical processes which have affected the evolution of mental health services is crucial if the mistakes of the past are to be avoided now that the government seems committed to renewed investment in residential mental health care.

If good-quality mental health care is to be developed in the future, it is important that people are not naïve about residential mental health care. Even after the worst features of the large psychiatric hospitals had been eliminated, they were not the ideal setting for caring for mentally distressed people. Indeed, while the years between the end of the Second World War and the early 1970s were character-ized by far-reaching and rapid social change, life inside many wards in Britain's psychiatric hospitals remained relatively unchanged (see Martin, 1984; Hopton, forthcoming). This was due to a combination of factors including chronic shortages of staff, a lack of systematic staff development, outdated buildings and the peculiar dynamics of the social organization of large institutions as described by Erving Goffman (see Beardshaw, 1981; Martin, 1984). Nevertheless, although their observations were later overshadowed by reports of corruption of care at several large psychiatric hospitals (see Martin, 1984), the committee which produced the 1968 Review of Psychiatric Nursing, *Psychiatric Nursing Today and Tomorrow*, identified some examples of good practice in such hospitals. However, as there was increasingly a shift towards community care and an emphasis on discharging all but the least capable long-stay hospital residents, the provision of democratic, user-centred residential care for mentally distressed individuals gradually became something of a lost art. If mental health policy is going to be based on the concept of increased residential care and better integration of residential and community-based services, there must be greater clarity about how residential services may be run on democratic and user-centred lines. Additionally, there is a need to consider how therapeutic interventions which might be offered in such settings might be different from, but of similar quality to, those offered to people living in 'the community'.

An important dimension to the history of mental health and mental distress is the emergence of competing ideologies of causation of and therapeutic responses to mental distress. There are so many of these that even the most dedicated full-time historian would have difficulty in identifying all of them and understanding their implications. Nevertheless, each perspective on mental distress and therapeutic intervention has its own internal logic. Therefore, the mental health professional who fails to acknowledge that there are so many alternatives is in danger of becoming a rigid dogmatist who is incapable of working in democratic and user-centred ways. Furthermore, simply knowing about other perspectives and being able to explore options with clients is not enough. There is no value in a mental health professional understanding the history of the policy and philosophy of mental health care unless s/he also appreciates the complex interaction of history, social structures, ideology and personal experience. In particular, it is important for mental health professionals to realize that mental distress may be more than a question of individual pathology. For example, it might be the product of discrimination, social exclusion or an exploitative relationship. In such circumstances, any therapeutic approach which emphasizes individual responsibility and/or the importance of adapting to circumstances would be more likely to compound a person's distress than help to alleviate it.

To summarize, embracing a critical perspective on mental health care requires commitment not only to helping the individual in distress, but also to identifying and eliminating the root causes of distress. Additionally, a mental health professional needs to be capable of negotiating care packages which are acceptable not only to each individual service user but also to that person's significant others, other members of the multi-disciplinary mental health care team and any other interested parties. To a certain extent all these issues are addressed in the existing literature on mental health, but the inter-relationship of these issues is rarely discussed. It is our contention that it is not possible to develop an integrated approach to mental health promotion and the alleviation of mental distress which is truly holistic, anti-oppressive, anti-discriminatory and therefore truly user-centred without consideration of this relationship. Furthermore, although it is beneficial to have a literature which addresses specific issues such as race, class, gender, institutional care, stigma and so on, the actual practice of mental health care should start from what is observed and reported, rather than from a theoretical premise. If there are issues arising from considerations such as gender, race or class which are pertinent to the situation of a mentally distressed person, they will emerge from dialogue with that person and others who are affected by that person's distress. In other words, the critically aware mental health professional should not attempt to impose an intellectual interpretation of a service user's problems on that person. To do so would be to run the risk of misinterpreting events, disregarding the service user's perceptions and overlooking real issues. For example, a mental health professional working from a theoretical perspective which defines racism only in terms of skin colour and/or neo-colonialism may overlook mental health problems which might be related to a sense of Welsh, Irish, Mediterranean or Jewish ethnic identity. Similarly, some radical feminist positions may lead someone to misunderstand or even trivialize forms of distress such as transsexual syndrome and gender dysphoria. Instead, mental health professionals should utilize their theoretical knowledge to help service users explore their circumstances and come to their own conclusions about why they are distressed and how they might overcome their problems.

The history of mental health services and research into mental distress shows that, despite years of research, there is not a universally accepted theory of mental health and mental distress. Consequently, the development of progressive mental health services has been hampered by the ideological struggles between the proponents of various different theoretical perspectives on mental health and mental distress. The perspectives which have hitherto gained prominence are almost exclusively those that emphasize individual pathology, whether it be biochemical, genetic or psychological and this is itself problematic. This is not to deny that such perspectives have made positive contributions to our understanding of mental distress and mental health. For example, it clearly is important for mental health professionals to be committed to expanding their self-awareness and developing their interpersonal skills. However, while such skills may be acquired through the systematic study of psychotherapeutic interventions, mental health care which is truly anti-oppressive, anti-discriminatory and user-centred cannot be based on therapy alone. There are situations where counselling, group or individual therapy, cognitive therapy and/or psychoactive medication may be of considerable benefit to an individual. Counselling may be beneficial if someone has had an unexpected bereavement; cognitive therapy may be an effective way of managing phobic anxiety; and psychoactive medication may be helpful as a short-term response to many acute forms of severe mental distress. However, there are situations where the causes of a person's distress are beyond their control and where conventional therapeutic responses are of limited value. For example, the problem may be inability to get access to material resources, daily experience of discrimination, social isolation or even a fundamental lack of self-confidence. In such cases, all conventional psychotherapy can offer is a new vocabulary for the person to express his/her unhappiness. Alternatively, medication would merely blunt a person's emotions so they would be less troubled by the misery of their experience, while all cognitive therapy could offer would be redefinition of the problem to make it appear less unpalatable.

David Cooper suggested that all mental distress is veiled political protest and that the role of the mental health professional should be to raise the political consciousness of the mentally distressed person and unite with him/her in political struggle against the sources of oppression. While this image of the mental health professional as a 'Robin Hood'-style leader of the downtrodden has a certain romantic appeal, it is highly problematic. First, mental distress is experienced by people from all strata of society, from people who are wealthy, privileged and powerful (for example, professional footballers, show-business personalities, politicians, members of royal families) through to people who are dispossessed, marginalized and powerless. Second, the two dominant British political trends of recent years – The New Right and New Labour – are based on notions of liberty and egalitarianism. Indeed, both ideologies have supporters and critics from diverse social and economic backgrounds. For example, it has often been suggested that the politics of the New Right appealed as much to working-class voters as it did to industrialists and financiers. Similarly, one of the most striking features of New Labour is its abandonment of traditional socialist values and its active recruitment of relatively prosperous middle-class professionals. Furthermore, despite Tony Blair's rhetoric of a third way, New Labour's concerns with 'stakeholding' and reducing social exclusion closely resemble the New Right idea that social justice for all will be achieved simply by creating mechanisms for consultation and equality of opportunity, rather than by engineering the redistribution of wealth. However, Cooper is not the only writer to acknowledge the connection between social and political circumstances and mental health. Other writers (notably Fanon and Reich, but also Fromm, Heimler and Frankl among others) have shown how experiences such as oppression, violent or sexual assault or social misfortune may have an impact on mental health. Such experiences may be ongoing and are shaped by forces beyond the control of the individual (for example, daily experience of discrimination or harassment) and/or are so traumatic that they cannot be redefined or forgotten (for example, surviving mass murder or child rape). In such cases conventional psychotherapy which promotes adaptation, and thereby implicitly discounts the practical and therapeutic value of direct action, is futile. Similarly, a mental health professional who is capable of nothing more than abstract intellectual or empathic understanding of a distressed person's circumstances is of limited usefulness in such circumstances. As Fanon argued, and Frankl and Heimler demonstrated by their own example, such individuals need to give meaning to their experiences, to reclaim their sense of self-worth and to take control of their own destiny. So-called therapeutic interventions which focus on reframing thoughts, adapting to circumstances and/or implicitly encouraging a person to think of themselves as victims of circumstance are likely to achieve the opposite. Furthermore, they have a tendency to foster feelings of dependency on the therapist as either a rescuer/saviour or bringer of enlightenment. By contrast, participation in collective endeavour (whether to build a community, participate in political struggle, raise funds for some kind of project or cause, develop a learning environment or create a work of art) facilitates the kind of self-discovery described by Fanon, Frankl, Heimler, Newman and others. Thus, the proper role of the enlightened mental health professional should not necessarily be the direct provision of therapy. It might equally be to assist someone to find and join a group or community to which they can make a positive contribution, and so give meaning to their own experience and discover their latent strengths and talents.

In conclusion, the role of the enlightened mental health professional would be a multi-faceted one, in which the role of personal therapist would be a relatively minor one. Certainly, mental health professionals will encounter individuals who require little more than short-term counselling and psychotherapy, while traditional psychotherapeutic skills may be needed in many crisis intervention scenarios or to support people through change. However, anti-psychiatry, sections of the mental health service users' movement, disillusioned psychotherapists such as Jeffrey Masson and others (notably Reich, Fanon and Newman) have highlighted the limitations of such approaches. Neither conventional psychotherapeutic approaches nor psychoactive drugs can address issues such as social isolation, alienation, exploitation, oppression and discrimination. Nevertheless, as such phenomena may contribute significantly to the development of an individual's mental distress, mental health professionals should be prepared to help service users address these problems. Accounts of various types of therapeutic community and of alternative communities such as communes and kibbutzim suggest that people who have had traumatic or unpleasant life experiences may derive various social and/or therapeutic benefits from joining such communities (see Bunker *et al.*, 1997; Kennard, 1998). Similarly, notwithstanding some of the controversies which surround his work at the East Side Institute for Short-Term Psychotherapy, Fred Newman's work there shows that participating in collective effort to sustain a particular community is therapeutic as it gives people a sense of being in control of their own destiny. Thus, an important role for the critically aware mental health professional would be to facilitate entry to such communities and/or to help people develop their own communities, so that community care might become a reality. The problem with the discourses of community care which have dominated mental health policy in recent years is that in late capitalist, post-industrial societies such as Britain, real communities based on an ethic of mutual care-giving and shared interest have become a comparative rarity – especially in urban areas. In this sense, community care has not failed as such because many people supposedly receiving care 'in the community' have remained socially isolated and alienated and have not therefore really belonged to a community.

If mental health care in the community is to become a reality, mental health professionals will need to undertake community development work. Although this sounds idealistic and over-ambitious, this need not involve trying to work up enthusiasm about community projects in a particular residential area. A community might as easily be based in a city-centre building which is either a permanent meeting place (not unlike Newman's East Side Institute), a place of residence or a combination of both as be centred on a housing estate or village. However, in such situations, care would have to be taken to ensure that there was permanent or semi-permanent membership, a shared sense of purpose, a spirit of co-operation, mutual interest and mutual concern so that such enterprises evolved into substantive communities and did not become casual 'drop-in' centres. Furthermore, such communities would need to be capable of providing 24-hour care and support to people experiencing acute crises of mental distress.

There would be several advantages to the primary focus of mental health care being community development rather than 'therapy'. First, whereas conventional therapies inevitably involve a therapist deliberately intervening with a service user, introducing someone to a community simply opens up a support network to the service user. If a service user is in crisis at the time of the introduction, such a support network might actively look after that person until the crisis subsides. When the crisis is past, or if the person joins the community before a crisis occurs or during a period of remission, there may be no uninvited intervention. The therapeutic value of being part of a community is rather that the person will gain a sense of purpose and self-worth from the contributions that s/he will be able to make to the collective life of the community. Second, the focus of being in a community is the potential positive contributions a person might make to collective endeavour rather than the real or perceived shortcomings and problems which are the focus of conventional therapy. Thus, theories of aetiology and pathology become relatively unimportant. Third, as communities are primarily settings for (mutual) care, rather than for the administration of treatments, severely distressed individuals need not fear or resist being introduced to them when they are experiencing a crisis. Fourth, while the administration of treatment is not the primary purpose of such a therapeutic community, neither need it be a taboo. A member of a community could, if s/he wished, receive any kind of treatment from counselling, through to the use of psychoactive drugs (or even electro-convulsive therapy or psychosurgery) without interfering with the ethos of the community. In essence, this would represent an integra-tion of some of the principles of therapeutic communities, the perspectives of the mental health service users' movement, the perspectives of critics of psychiatry and psychotherapy and more conventional responses to mental distress.

Experiments such as Kingsley Hall, The Richmond Fellowship, the Arbours and Philadelphia Associations (see Kennard, 1998) and the apparent success of the East Side Institute of Short-Term Psychother-apy indicate that this is no mere pipe dream. On the other hand, such enterprises have chosen to remain separate from the mainstream and self-consciously represent an alternative to conventional therapy. If they had not adopted such a strategy, their ideals may well have been compromised, and we would not be able to identify them as relatively successful experiments in alternative approaches to the management of mental distress. On the other hand, those associated with such experiments have tended to dogmatically reject therapeutic interven-tions to which they have ideological objections. At the present time the two main driving forces behind the formulation of mental health policy are responsiveness to the needs and wishes of service users and belief in the importance of evidence-based practice. The logic of both these imperatives dictates that while there is evidence that some kind of community development (i.e. the success of The Richmond Fellow-ship, Arbours and Philadelphia Associations etc.) is an important dimension to mental health care, it is only one of several important dimensions. There is also evidence that counselling, psychotherapy, psychoactive medication and even ECT may be effective responses to certain forms of mental distress in certain circumstances and that some service users will willingly accept such treatments (see Perkins, 1999b). Consequently, skills in community development and the brokerage of care packages should be seen as skills which mental health professionals need to develop alongside the skills and knowl-edge traditionally associated with their work.

In short, community development alone is never going to be an absolute answer to the problems posed by mental distress. However, it does represent a starting point for a form of mental health care which is sensitive to the needs of mentally distressed persons, and the needs of those who may themselves be disturbed by the behaviour of people experiencing acute distress. It is an approach which can accommodate most perspectives on mental distress whether they be socio-political, psychiatric, psychotherapeutic or reflect a discourse of anti-therapy.

Bibliography

Abel, K., Buszewicz, M., Davison, S., Johnson, S. and Staples, E. (Eds) (1996) *Planning Mental Health Services for Women: a Multiprofessional Handbook*, London, Routledge.

Abercrombie, N., Hill, S. and Turner, B. S. (1988) *Dictionary of Sociology*, London, Penguin.

Ackner, B. (1964) *Handbook for Psychiatric Nurses*, London, Bailliere Tindall.

Ackroyd, C., Margolis, K., Rosenhead, J. and Shallice, T. (1980) *The Technology of Political Control*, London, Pluto.

Ahmad, W. (Ed.) (1993) *'Race' and Health in Contemporary Britain*, Buckingham, Open University Press.

Ahmed, T. and Webb-Johnson, A. (1995) 'Voluntary groups', in Fernando, S. (Ed.) *Mental Health in a Multi-ethnic Society: A Multi-disciplinary Handbook*, London, Routledge.

Allen, H. (1986) 'Psychiatry and the construction of the feminine', in Miller, P. and Rose, N. (Eds) *The Power of Psychiatry*, Cambridge, Polity Press.

American Psychiatric Association (1994) *Diagnostic and Statistical Manual of Mental Disorders*, 4th Edition (DSM IV), Washington, American Psychiatric Association.

Anderson, E. W. and Trethowan, W. H. (1973) *Psychiatry*, London, Bailliere Tindall.

Andrews, J., Briggs, A., Porter, R., Tucker, P. and Waddington, K. (1997) *The History of Bedlam*, London, Routledge.

Andrews, M. (1988) 'Changing disruptive behaviour in an adult training centre client', *Behavioural Psychotherapy*, **16** (2), pp. 108–114.

Audit Commission (1986) *Making a Reality of Community Care*, London, HMSO.

Audit Commission (1994) *Finding a Place*, London, HMSO.

Baker, P. (1993) 'The British Experience', in Romme, M. and Escher, S. *Accepting Voices*, London, MIND.

Ballard, J. (1994) 'District nurses: who's looking after them?', *Occupational Health Review*, November/December i–x.

Ballard, R. (1979) 'Ethnic minorities and the social services' in Khan, V. S. (Ed.) *Minority Families in Britain: Support and Stress*, London, Macmillan.

Bandler, R. and Grinder, J. (1982) *Re-framing: Neuro-linguistic Programming*™ *and the Transformation of Meaning*, Moab, Real People Press.

Barker, M. (1981) *The New Racism* London, Junction Books.

Barnes, D. M. (1987) 'Biological issues in schizophrenia', *Science*, **235**, pp. 430–433.

Barrett, M. and Roberts, H. (1978) 'Doctors and their patients', in Smart, H. and Smart, B. (Eds) *Women, Sexuality and Social Control*, London, Routledge and Kegan Paul.

Barton, W. R. (1959) *Institutional Neurosis*, Bristol, Wright and Sons.

Baruch, G. and Treacher, A. (1978) *Psychiatry Observed*, London, Routledge and Kegan Paul.

Batchelor, I. (1969) *Henderson & Gillespie's Textbook of Psychiatry*, Oxford, Oxford University Press.

Bateson, G. (1962) *Perceval's Narrative: A Patient's Account of his Psychosis 1830–1832*, London, Hogarth Press.

Bean, P. (1980) *Compulsory Admissions to Mental Hospital*, Chichester, Wiley.

Beardshaw, V. (1981) *Conscientious Objectors at Work*, London Social Audit.

Beck, A. T. (1967) *Depression: Causes and Treatment*, Philadelphia, University of Pennsylvania Press.

Becker, H. (1963) *Outsiders*, New York, Free Press.

Beliappa, J. (1991) *Illness or Distress? Alternative Models of Mental Health*, London, Confederation of Indian Organisations.

Bentall, R. P. (Ed.) (1992) *Reconstructing Schizophrenia*, London, Routledge.

Bergin, A. and Lambert, M. (1978) 'The evaluation of therapeutic outcomes', in Garfield, S. and Bergin, A. (Eds) *Handbook of Psychotherapy and Behaviour Change*, 2nd Edition, Chichester, Wiley.

Bergin, A.E. (1971) 'The evaluation of therapeutic outcomes', in Bergin, A. E. and Garfield, S. (Eds) *Handbook of Psychotherapy and Behaviour Change*, New York, Wiley.

Berke, J. (1969) *Counter Culture*, London, Peter Owen Ltd.

Berke, J. H. (1979) *I Haven't Had to Go Mad Here*, Harmondsworth, Penguin.

Berke, J. H. (1997) Telephone conversation with John Hopton, 25 May.

Berke, J. H., Masoliver, C. and Ryan, T. J. (1995) *Sanctuary*, London, Process Press.

Berne, E. (1968) *Games People Play*, Harmondsworth, Penguin.

Berne, E. (1975) *What Do You Say After You Say Hello?*, London, Corgi.

Berrios, G. and Freeman, H. (1991) *One Hundred and Fifty Years of British Psychiatry 1841–1991*, London, Royal College of Psychiatrists/Gaskell.

Bettelheim, B. (1986) *The Informed Heart*, London, Peregrine.

Bigwood, L. (1990) 'Lyn Bigwood, RMN talks to R.D. Laing – Sanity, Madness and the Psychiatric Profession', *Asylum*, **4** (2), pp. 18–31.

Birke, L. (1986) *Women, Feminism and Biology*, Brighton, Wheatsheaf.

Blackburn, C. (1991) *Poverty and Health – Working with Families*, Buckingham, Open University Press.

Blom-Cooper, L. (1992) *Report of the Committee of Inquiry into Ashworth Hospital*, London, HMSO.

Blom-Cooper, L., Hally, H. and Murphy, E. (1995) *The Falling Shadow: One Patient's Mental Health Care 1978–1993*, London, Duckworth.

Bolton, P. (1984) 'Management of compulsorily admitted patients to a high security unit', *International Journal of Social Psychiatry*, **30**, pp. 77–84.

Bott, E. (1975) 'Hospital and Society', *British Journal of Medical Psychology*, **49**, pp. 97–140.

Boyle, M. (1993) *Schizophrenia: a Scientific Delusion?*, London, Routledge.

Bracken, P. J., Greenslade, L., Griffin, B. and Smyth, M. (1998) 'Mental health and ethnicity: an Irish dimension', *British Journal of Psychiatry*, **172**, pp. 103–105.

Braid, M. (1995) 'Send in the counsellors', *The Independent (Section Two)*, 13 December, pp. 6–7.

Breggin, P. (1973) 'The final solution: the killing of mental patients', *Freedom – The Independent Journal of the Church of Scientology*, June/July, pp. 5–7 (reprinted in *Asylum*, **6** (2), pp. 24–26, 1992).

Breggin, P. (1979) *Electroshock: Its Brain-disabling Effects*, New York, Springer.

Breggin, P. (1993) *Toxic Psychiatry*, London, HarperCollins.

Briscoe, M. (1982) 'Sex differences in psychological wellbeing', *Psychological Medicine*, Monographs, Supplement 1.

Broad, C. D. (1962) *Lectures on Psychical Research*, London, Routledge and Kegan Paul.

Broadhurst, D. (1997) *The History of Parkside Hospital, Macclesfield 1841–1996: A Sense of Perspective*, Leek, Churnet Valley Books.

Broverman, I. K., Broverman, D. M., Clarkson, F. E., Rosenkrantz, P. S. and Vogel, S. R. (1970) 'Sex role stereotypes and clinical judgement of mental health', *Journal of Consulting and Clinical Psychology*, **34**, pp. 1–7.

Brown, G. W. (1959) 'Experiences of discharged chronic schizophrenic patients in various types of living group', *Millbank Memorial Fund Quarterly*, **37**, p. 105.

Brown, G. W. and Harris, T. (1978) *Social Origins of Depression*, London, Tavistock.

Brown, G. W. and Wing, J. K. (1962) 'A comparative clinical and social survey of three mental hospitals', *The Sociological Review Monograph*, **5**, pp. 145–171.

Browne, D. (1995) *An Element of Compulsion*, London, Commission for Racial Equality.

Bryan, B., Dadzie, S. and Scafe, S. (1985) *The Heart of the Race: Black Women's Lives in Britain*, London, Virago.

Buchan, H. *et al.* (1992) 'Who benefits from electroconvulsive therapy? Combined results of the Leicester and Northwick Park trials', *British Journal of Psychiatry*, **160**, pp. 355–359.

Bunker, S., Coates, C., How, J., Jones, L. and Morris, W. (Eds) (1997) *Diggers & Dreamers: The Guide to Communal Living 98/99*, London, Diggers and Dreamers Publications.

Burke, A. W. (1984) 'Racism and mental illness', *International Journal of Social Psychiatry*, 30th Anniversary Double Issue.

Burleigh, M. (1994) *Death and Deliverance: Euthanasia in Germany c1900-1945*, Cambridge, Cambridge University Press.

Burnham, M. A. *et al.* (1988) *Journal of Consulting and Clinical Psychology*, **56**, pp. 843–850.

Busfield, J. (1986) *Managing Madness: Changing Ideas and Practice*, London, Hutchinson.

Busfield, J. (1996) *Men, Women and Madness: Understanding Gender and Mental Disorder*, London, Macmillan.

Bynum, W. F., Porter, R. and Shepherd, M. (Eds) (1985a) *The Anatomy of Madness: Essays in the History of Psychiatry*, Volume 1, London, Tavistock.

Bynum, W. F., Porter, R. and Shepherd, M. (Eds) (1985b) *The Anatomy of Madness: Essays in the History of Psychiatry*, Volume 2, London, Tavistock.

Bynum, W. F., Porter, R. and Shepherd, M. (Eds) (1988) *The Anatomy of Madness: Essays in the History of Psychiatry*, Volume 3, London, Tavistock.

Calabrese, J. R. and Markovitz, P. J. (1991) 'Treatment of depression. New pharmacologic approaches', *Primary Care*, **18** (2), pp. 421–433.

Campbell, P. (1989) 'Peter Campbell's Story', in Brackx, A. and Grimshaw, C. (Eds) *Mental Health Care in Crisis*, London, Pluto.

Campbell, P. (1991) 'The User Movement', *Oxford Survivors Libellus Dementum*, **1** (1), pp. 4–12.

Campling, P. and Haigh, R. (1999) *Therapeutic Communities Past, Present and Future*, London, Jessica Kinglsey.

Caplan, P. J., McMurdy-Myers, J. and Gans, M. (1992) 'Should "premenstrual syndrome" be called a psychiatric abnormality?', *Feminism and Psychology*, **2** (1), pp. 27–44.

Capra, F. (1983) *The Turning Point*, London, Flamingo.

Carpenter, I. and Brockington, I. (1980) 'A study of mental illness in Asians, West Indians and Africans living in Manchester', *British Journal of Psychiatry*, **137**, pp. 201–205.

Castel, R. (1976) *The Regulation of Madness: Origins of Incarceration in France*, Oxford, Polity Press.

Chakrabarti, M. (1990) 'Racial Prejudice', *Open University Workbook 6, Part 1 of K254 Working with Children and Young People*, Milton Keynes, Open University.

Chamberlain, J. (1988) *On Our Own – Patient-controlled Alternatives to the Mental Health System*, London, MIND.

Charlton, B. (1998) 'Life before health', in Anderson, D. and Mullen, P. (Eds) *Faking It*, London, The Social Affairs Unit.

Chen, E. Y. H., Harrison, G. and Standen, P. J. (1991) 'Management of first episode psychotic illness in Afro-Caribbean patients', *British Journal of Psychiatry*, **158**, pp. 517–522.

Chesler, P. (1972) *Women and Madness*, New York, Doubleday.

Chesler, P. (1990) 'Twenty years since *Women and Madness*: toward a feminist institute of mental health and healing', in Cohen, D. (Ed.) *Challenging the Therapeutic State: Critical Perspectives on Psychiatry and the Mental Health System*, Institute of Mind and Behaviour.

Chodorow, N. (1978) *The Reproduction of Mothering: Psychoanalysis and the Sociology of Gender*, California, University of California Press.

Ciompi, L. (1982) 'Is there really a schizophrenia?: the long term course of psychotic phenomena', *British Journal of Psychiatry*, **145**, pp. 636–640.

Clare, A. (1976) *Psychiatry in Dissent: Controversial Issues in Thought and Practice*, London, Tavistock.

Clark, D. (1996) *The Story of a Mental Hospital – Fulbourn 1858–1983*, London, Process Press.

Clark, D. H. (1974) *Social Therapy in Psychiatry*, Harmondsworth, Penguin.

Clarke, J. and Newman, J. (1997) *The Managerial State*, London, Sage.

Clarke, P.D. (1994) *Human Rights and the 'Mental Health' System*, unpublished MA Thesis, Edge Hill College of Higher Education.

Clayton, W. T. (1981) 'The use of positive reinforcement and stimulus fading in the treatment of an elective mute', *Behavioural Psychotherapy*, **9** (1), pp. 25–33.

Cobb, A. (1993) *Safe and Effective? MIND's Views on Psychiatric Drugs, ECT and Psychosurgery*, London, MIND.

Cochrane, R. (1977) 'Mental illness in immigrants to England and Wales: an analysis of mental hospital admissions 1971', *Social Psychiatry*, **12**, pp. 2–35.

Cochrane, R. and Bal, S. (1989) 'Mental hospital admission rates of immigrants to England: a comparison of 1971 and 1981', *Social Psychiatry*, **24**, pp. 2–11.

Cohen, D. (1989) *Soviet Psychiatry*, London, Paladin.

Cohen, D. (Ed.) (1990) *Challenging the Therapeutic State: Perspectives on Psychiatry and the Mental Health System*, Institute of Mind and Behaviour.

Cohen, S. and Scull, A. (Eds) (1983) *Social Control and the State*, Oxford, Blackwell.

Cohn, H. (1997) *Existential Thought and Therapeutic Practice: An Introduction to Existential Psychotherapy*, London, Sage.

Coleman, R. (1996/1997) 'The politics of the illness', *Asylum*, **10** (1), pp. 11–15.

Commission for Racial Equality (1992) *Race Relations Code of Practice: for the elimination of racial discrimination and the promotion of equal opportunity in the provision of mental health services*, London, Commission for Racial Equality.

Conran, M. (1986) 'The patient in hospital', *Psychoanalytic Psychotherapy*, **1** (1), pp. 31–43.

Conran, M. (1997) Interview with John Hopton, 24 June. Tape and transcript held by Planned Environment Therapy Trust, Church Lane, Toddington, Cheltenham GL54 5DQ.

Cook, J. and Marshall, J. (1996) 'Homeless women', in Abel, K. *et al.* (Eds)

Planning Community Mental Health Services for Women, London, Routledge.

Cooper, D. (1968) (Ed.) *The Dialectics of Liberation*, Harmondsworth, Pelican.

Cooper, D. (1970) *Psychiatry and Anti-psychiatry*, St Albans, Paladin.

Cooper, D. (1972) *The Death of the Family*, Harmondsworth, Pelican.

Cooper, D. (1976) *The Grammar of Living*, Harmondswoth, Pelican.

Cooper, D. (1980) *The Language of Madness*, Harmondsworth, Pelican.

Cooper, J. and Lewis, J. (1995) *Who Can I Talk to? The User's Guide to Therapy and Counselling*, London, Headway.

Cooper, R., Friedman, J., Gans, S., Heaton, J., Oakley, C., Oakley, H. and Zeal, P. (1989) *Thresholds Between Philosophy and Psychoanalysis*, London, Free Association Books.

Cooperstock, R. (1981) 'A Review of Women's Psychotropic Drug Use', in Howell, E. and Bayes, M. (Eds) *Women and Mental Health*, New York, Basic Books.

Cope, R. (1989) 'The compulsory detention of Afro-Caribbeans under the Mental Health Act', *New Community*, **15** (3), pp. 343–356.

Cornwell, J. (1984) *Hard-earned Lives: Accounts of Health and Illness in East London*, London, Tavistock.

Corob, A. (1987) *Working with Depressed Women*, Aldershot, Gower.

Coulshed, V. (1988) *Social Work Practice: An Introduction*, Basingstoke, Macmillan.

Coward, R. (1984) *Female Desire: Women's Sexuality Today*, London, Paladin.

Cox, T. (1996) 'Introducing NLP', <http://www.hollis.co.uk/jsa/>, Accessed July 1998.

Craib, I. (1992) *Modern Social Theory: From Parsons to Habermas*, 2nd Edition, London, Harvester Wheatsheaf.

Crepaz-Keay, D. (1998) 'The vision thing', *OpenMind*, **93**, p. 6.

Crossley, N. (1998) 'R. D. Laing and the British Anti-psychiatry Movement: A Socio-Historical Analysis', *Social Science and Medicine*, **47** (7), pp. 877–889.

Crotty, M. (1998) *The Foundations of Social Research: Meaning and Perspective in the Research Process*, London, Sage.

Curreen, M. P. (1996) 'A simple hypnotically based NLP technique used with two clients in criminal justice settings', *Australian Journal of Clinical and Experimental Hypnosis*, **24** (1), pp. 51–57.

Daly, M. (1979) *Gyn/Ecology: the metaethics of radical feminism*, London, The Women's Press.

Davidge, M., Elias, S., Jayes, B., Wood, K. and Yates, J. (1993) *Survey of English Mental Illness Hospitals*, University of Birmingham: Inter-Authority Comparisons and Consultancy Health Services Management Centre.

Davidson, V. (1984) 'Psychiatry's problem with no name: therapist-patient sex', in Reiker, P. and Carmen, E. (Eds) *The Gender Gap in Psychotherapy*, New York, Plenum Press.

Davies, D. and Neal, C. (Eds) (1996) *Pink Therapy*, Milton Keynes, Open University Press.

De Beauvoir, S. (1972) *The Second Sex*, Harmondsworth, Penguin.

De Swaan, A. (1990) *The Management of Normality*, London, Routledge.

Dean, G., Walsh, D., Downing, H. and Shelly, P. (1981) 'First admission of native-born and immigrants to psychiatric hospitals in South-East England 1976', *British Journal of Psychiatry*, **139**, pp. 506–512.

Department of Health (1989) *Caring for People: Community Care in the Next Decade and Beyond*, Cm 849, London, HMSO.

Department of Health (1994a) *Review of Health and Social Services for Mentally Disordered Offenders and Others Requiring Similar Services*, London, HMSO.

Department of Health (1994b) *Mental Health Task Force, Local Systems of Support: A Framework for Purchasing for People with Severe Mental Health Problems*, London, HMSO.

Department of Health (1996) *Report of the Confidential Inquiry into Homicides and Suicides by Mentally Ill People*, London, HMSO.

Department of Health (1998) *Modernising Mental Health Services: Safe, Sound and Supportive*, London, HMSO.

Department of Health (1999) *The Report of the Committee of Inquiry into the Personality Disorder Unit, Ashworth Special Hospital*, Cm 4195, London, HMSO.

Department of Health /Special Health Services Authority (1992) *Report of the Committee of Inquiry into Complaints about Ashworth Hospital*, Cmd 2028-1, London, HMSO.

Digby, A. (1985) *Moral Treatment at the Retreat 1796–1914*, Cambridge, Cambridge University Press.

Dinnerstein, D. (1976) *The Mermaid and the Minotaur: Sexual Arrangements and the Human Malaise*, New York, Harper and Row.

Dobash, R. E. and Dobash, R. (1979) *Violence Against Wives: A Case Against the Patriarchy*, New York, Free Press.

Doerner, K. (1981) *Madmen and the Bourgeoisie*, Oxford, Basil Blackwell.

Dohrenwend, B. P. and Dohrenwend, B. S. (1969) *Social Status and Psychological Disorders: A Casual Inquiry*, London, Wiley.

Dominelli, L. (1988) *Anti-racist Social Work*, London, Macmillan.

Donovan, J. (1986) 'We don't buy sickness, it just comes', *Health, Illness and Health Care in the Lives of Black People in London*, Aldershot, Gower.

Donzelot, J. (1980) *The Policing of Families*, London, Hutchinson.

Double, D. B. (1992) 'Training in Anti-psychiatry', *Asylum*, **6** (2), pp. 15–16.

Doyal, L. (1979) *The Political Economy of Health*, London, Pluto.

Drake, R. E. and Ehrlich, J. (1985) 'Suicide attempts associated with akathesia' *American Journal of Psychiatry*, **120**, pp. 151–154.

Dyer, C. (1994) 'Sad story of the happy pills' *The Guardian*, 10 May, p. 21.

Edwards, S. (1988) 'Mad, bad or pre-menstrual?', *New Law Journal*, **138**(6363).

Egan, G. (1994) *The Skilled Helper*, Pacific Grove, CA, Brooks Cole.

Ehrenreich, B. and English, D. (1974) *Witches, midwifery and nurses: a history of women healers*, London, Compendium.

Ehrenreich, B. and English, D. (1976) *Complaints and Disorders: The Sexual Politics of Sickness*, London, Writers and Readers Publishing Cooperative.

Ehrenreich, B. and English, D. (1979) *For Her Own Good: One Hundred and Fifty Years of the Experts' Advice to Women*, New York, Anchor Press.

Eichenbaum, L. and Orbach, S. (1982) *Outside In … Inside Out: Women's Psychology, a Feminist Psychoanalytic Approach*, Harmondsworth, Penguin.

Eichenbaum, L. and Orbach, S. (1984) *What Do Women Want?*, London, Fontana.

Ellenberger, H. (1970) *The Discovery of the Unconscious: The History and Evolution of Dynamic Psychiatry*, London, Allen Lane.

Ellis, A. (1962) *Reason and Emotion in Psychotherapy*, New York, Lyle Stuart.

Ernst, S. and Goodison, L. (1981) *In Our Own Hands: A Book of Self-help Therapy*, London, Women's Press.

Ettore, E. and Riska, E. (1993) 'Psychotropics, sociology and women', *Sociology of Health and Illness*, **15**, pp. 503–524.

Ewins, D. (1974) *The Origins of the Compulsory Commitment Provisions of the Mental Health Act (1959)*, unpublished MA Thesis, University of Sheffield.

Eysenck, H. J. (1952) 'The effects of psychotherapy, an evaluation', *Journal of Consulting Psychology*, **16**, pp. 319–324.

Eysenck, H. J. (1965) 'The effects of psychotherapy', *International Journal of Psychiatry*, **1**, pp. 99–144.

Fanon, F. (1967) *The Wretched of the Earth*, Harmondsworth, Penguin.

Fanon, F. (1986) *Black Skin, White Masks*, London, Pluto.

Farmer, A. and Owen, M. J. (1996) 'Genomics: the next psychiatric revolution?', *British Journal of Psychiatry*, **169** (2), pp. 135–138.

Farrell, E. (1991) *The Mental Health Survival Guide*, London, Optima.

Fennell, P. (1996) *Treatment Without Consent*, London, Routledge.

Fenton, S. and Sadiq, A. (1991) *Asian Women and Depression*, London, Commission for Racial Equality.

Fernando, S. (1986) 'Depression in ethnic minorities', in Cox, J. L. (Ed.) *Transcultural Psychiatry*, London, Croom Helm.

Fernando, S. (1988) *Race and Culture in Psychiatry*, London, Croom Helm.

Fernando, S. (1991) *Mental Health, Race and Culture*, London, Macmillan.

Fernando, S. (1992) 'Roots of Racism in Psychiatry', *OpenMind*, **59**, pp. 10–11.

Fernando, S. (Ed.) (1995) *Mental Health in a Multi-ethnic Society: A Multi-disciplinary Handbook*, London, Routledge.

Ferns, P. and Madden, M. (1995) 'Training to provide race equality', in Fernando, S. (Ed.) *Mental Health in a Multi-ethnic Society: A Multi-disciplinary Handbook*, London, Routledge.

Finch, J. and Groves, D. L. (Eds) (1983) *A Labour of Love: Women, Work and Caring*, London, Routledge.

Finch, J. and Mason, D. (1992) *Negotiating Family Responsibilities*, London, Routledge.

Fordham, F. (1966) *An Introduction to Jung's Psychology*, Harmondsworth, Pelican.

Foucault, M. (1967) *Madness and Civilisation*, London, Tavistock.

Foucault, M. (1972) *The Archaeology of Knowledge*, New York, Harper and Row.

Foucault, M. (1977) *Discipline and Punish: The Birth of the Prison*, London, Allen Lane.

Foucault, M. (1980) *Power/Knowledge: Selected Interviews and Other Writings 1972–1977*, Brighton, Harvester Press.

Francis, E. (1989) 'Black people, dangerousness and psychiatric compulsion', in Brackx, A. and Grimshaw, C. (Eds) *Mental Health Care in Crisis*, London, Pluto.

Francis, E. (1991) 'Mental health, anti-racism and social work training', in CCETSW (Ed.) *One Small Step Towards Racial Justice*, London, CCETSW.

Francis, E. (1996) 'Community care, danger and black people', in *Open Mind*, **80**, April/May, pp. 4–5.

Frankl, V. E. (1984) *Man's Search for Meaning*, New York, Washington Square Press.

Franklin, B. and Parton, N. (1991) *Social Work, Media and Public Relations*, London, Routledge.

Fraser, D., Anderson J. and Grime, J. (1981) 'An analysis of the progressive development of vocal responses in a mute schizophrenic patient', *Behavioural Psychotherapy*, **9** (1), pp. 2–12.

Freud, S. (1953) *A General Introduction to Psychoanalysis*, New York, Liveright/Pocket Books.

Friedan, B. (1963) *The Feminine Mystique*, Harmondsworth, Penguin.

Fromm, E. (1979) *To Have or To Be*, London, Abacus.

Fromm, E. (1990) *Man for Himself*, London, Routledge.

Galton, F. (1869) *Hereditary Genius*, London, Macmillan.

Galton, F. (1889) *Natural Inheritance*, London and New York, Macmillan.

Gilroy, P. (1993) 'One nation under a groove', in *Small Acts. Thoughts on the Politics of Black Cultures*, London, Serpent's Tail.

Gittins, D. (1998a) *Madness in its Place: Narratives of Severalls Hospital 1913–1997*, London, Routledge.

Gittins, D. (1998b) 'When the Walls Came Down', *Community Care*, 21–27 May.

Goddard, J. (1996) *Mixed Feelings: Littlemore Hospital – An Oral History Project*, Oxford, Oxfordshire County Council.

Goffman, E. (1961) *Asylums: Essays on the Social Situation of Mental Patients and Other Inmates*, Harmondsworth, Penguin.

Goldberg, D. and Huxley, P (1980) *Mental Illness in the Community: The Pathways to Psychiatric Care*, London, Tavistock.

Gostin, L. O. (1975) *A Human Condition*, Volume 1, London, National Association for Mental Health.

Gostin, L. O. (1977) *A Human Condition*, Volume 2, London, National Association for Mental Health.

Goulding, R. A. and Schwartz, R. C. (1995) *The Mosaic Mind*, New York, W.W. Norton.

Gove, W. (1979) 'Sex differences in the epidemiology of mental illness: evidence and explanations', in Gomberg, E. and Franks, V. (Eds) *Gender and Disordered Behaviour*, New York, Brunner/Mazel.

Graham, H. (1993) *Hardship and Health in Women's Lives*, Hemel Hempstead, Harvester Wheatsheaf.

Grant, G. (1995) 'Assessment and care management: a service sector view', *Centre for Social Policy and Research Newsletter*, Summer, pp. 5–12, University of Wales, Bangor, CSPRD.

Grant, L. (1992) 'Counselling: a solution ... or a problem?' *The Independent on Sunday*, 19 April, pp. 22–23.

Green, D. G. (1987) *The New Right*, Brighton, Wheatsheaf.

Greenberg, R. P., Bornstein, R. F., Zborowski, M. J., Fisher, S. and Greenberg, M. D. (1994) 'A meta-analysis of fluoexetine outcome in the treatment of depression', *Journal of Nervous and Mental Disorder*, **182** (10), pp. 547–551.

Greenslade, L. (1994) 'Caoinean an Ion dubh: towards an Irish dimension in 'ethnic' health', *Irish Studies Review*, **8**, pp. 2–5.

Grierson, M. (1991) *A Report of the Manchester Hearing Voices Conference*, Manchester, Hearing Voices Network.

Griffiths, Sir R. (1988) *Community Care: An Agenda for Action*, London, HMSO.

Griggs, C. (1998) *S/he: Changing Sex and Changing Clothes*, Berg Publishing.

Grinder, J. and Bandler, R. (1981) *Trance-formations: Neuro-linguistic Programming and the Structure of Hypnosis*, Moab, Real People Press.

Guimon, J. (1989) 'The Biases of psychiatric diagnosis', *British Journal of Psychiatry*, Supplement 4, pp. 33–37.

Haddock, G. and Slade, P. D. (1996) *Cognitive-behavioural Interventions with Psychotic Disorders*, London, Routledge.

Hadley, R. and Clough, R. (1997) *Care in Chaos: Frustration and Challenge in Community Care*, London, Cassell.

Hall, J. N. and Rosenthal, G. (1973) 'Operant treatment of the long-term patient', in Nursing Times Services, *The Psychiatric Nurse as Therapist*, London, Macmillan Journals, pp. 8–14.

Harding, T. W. (1990) ' "Not Worth Powder and Shot" – A Reappraisal of Montagu Lomax's Contribution to Mental Health Reform', *British Journal of Psychiatry*, **156**, pp. 180–187.

Harris, T. A. (1973) *I'm OK – You're OK*, London, Pan.

Harris, V. (1995) 'Unwanted inheritance', *Community Care*, 23 February–1 March.

Harrison, D. (1995) *Vicious Circles*, London, Good Practices in Mental Health.

Harrison, G., Owens, D., Holton, A., Neilson, D., and Boot, D. (1988) 'A prospective study of severe mental disorder in Afro-Caribbean patients', *Psychological Medicine*, **11**, pp. 289–302.

Haughton, P. and Sawa, T. (1993) *Black Perspectives in the Voluntary Sector*, London, Thames/LWT Telethon Report.

Healy, D. (1990a) 'The psychopharmacological era: notes toward a history', *Journal of Psychopharmacology*, **4**, pp. 152–167.

Healy, D. (1990b) *The Suspended Revolution*, London, Faber and Faber.

Healy, D. (1991) 'D1 and D2 and D3', *British Journal of Psychiatry*, **159**, pp. 319–324.

Healy, D., Savage, M. and Thomas, P. (1998) Abusive prescribing, *OpenMind*, **93**, pp. 8–9.

Hedaya, R. J. (1996) *Understanding Biological Psychiatry*, New York, W. W. Norton.

Heimler, E. (1962) *A Link in the Chain*, London, The Bodley Head.

Heimler, E. (1967) *Mental Illness and Social Work*, Harmondsworth, Penguin.

Henwood, M. (1994) *Fit for Change? Snapshots of the Community Care Reforms One Year On*, London, King's Fund Centre.

Herman, D. and Green, J. (1991) *Madness: A Study Guide*, London, BBC/Mental Health Media Council.

Herrnstein, R. J. and Murray, C. (1994) *The Bell Curve: Intelligence and Class Structure in American Life*, New York, Free Press.

Hinchliffe, M. (1991) 'Socialism and mental health', *Asylum*, **5** (1), pp. 12–16.

Hinchliffe, M. (1995) 'Haunted Houses: R. D. Laing – A Biography by Adrian Laing', *Asylum*, **9** (1), pp. 37–39.

Hinds, A. (1992) *Report on Organisations Serving the Afro-Caribbean Community*, London, West Indian Standing Conference.

Hitch, P. (1981) 'Immigration and mental health: local research and social explanations' *New Community*, **9**, pp. 256–262.

HMSO (1980) *Behaviour Modification*, London, HMSO.

Holland, S. (1990) 'Psychotherapy, oppression and social action: gender, race and class in black women's depression', in Perelberg, R. J. and Miller, A. C. (Eds) *Gender and Power in Families*, London, Routledge.

Holland, S. (1992) 'From social abuse to social action: a neighbourhood psycho-therapy and social action programme for women', in Ussher, J. M. and Nicolson, P. (Eds) *Gender Issues in Clinical Psychology*, London, Routledge.

Holland, S. (1995) 'Interaction in women's mental health and neighbourhood development', in Fernando, S. (Ed.) *Mental Health in a Multi-ethnic Society: A Multi-disciplinary Handbook*, London, Routledge.

Hopton, J. (1994/95) 'User involvement in the education of mental health nurses. An evaluation of possibilities', *Critical Social Policy*, **42**, Winter, pp. 47–62.

Hopton, J. (1995) 'Control and restraint in contemporary psychiatric nursing: some clinical considerations', *Journal of Advanced Nursing*, **22**, pp. 110–115.

Hopton, J. (1997a) 'Towards a critical theory of mental health nursing', *Journal of Advanced Nursing*, **25** (3), pp. 492–500.

Hopton, J. (1997b) 'Who are we listening to?' *Nursing Times*, **93** (41), pp. 44–45.

Hopton, J. (1998) 'Risk assessment using psychological profiling techniques: an evaluation of possibilities', *British Journal of Social Work*, **28**, pp. 247–261.

Hopton, J. (1999) 'Prestwich Hospital in the twentieth century: a case study of slow and uneven progress in the development of psychiatric care', *History of Psychiatry*, **10** (3), pp. 349–369.

Hopton, J. and Glenister, D. (1996) 'Working in partnership: vision or pipe dream?', *Critical Social Policy*, **16** (2), pp. 111–120.

Hospital Doctor (1995) 'Why consultants want out', 14 September, p. 7.

House of Commons Health Select Committee (1994) *Better Off in the Community? The Care of People Who Are Seriously Mentally Ill*, London, HMSO.

House of Commons Social Services Committee (1985) *Community Care with Special Reference to Adult Mentally Ill and Mentally Handicapped People*, London, HMSO.

House, R. (1996) 'Psychotherapy and counselling on the run', *Asylum*, **9** (4), pp. 33–35.

Houston, G. (1982) *The Red Book of Gestalt*, London, Rochester Foundation.

Hugman, R. (1991) *Power in Caring Professions*, Basingstoke, Macmillan.

Hunter, D. (1992) 'The move to community care with special reference to mental illness', in Beck, E. *et al.* (Eds) *In the Best of Health*, London, Chapman and Hall.

Hunter, P. and Kelso, E. (1985) 'Feminist behaviour therapy', *Behaviour Therapist*, **8** (10), pp. 201–204.

Hunter, R. and MacAlpine, I. (1963) *Three Hundred Years of Psychiatry, 1535 to 1860: A History Presented in Selected English Texts*, London, Oxford University Press.

Husband, C. (1994) *'Race' and the Nation: The British Experience*, Curtin University of Technology, Bentley, Western Australia, Paradigm Books.

Illich, I. (1975) *Medical Nemesis*, London, Calder and Boyars.

Illich, I. (1976) *Limits to Medicine*, Harmondsworth, Penguin.

Ineichen, B. (1986) 'Compulsory admission to psychiatric hospital under the 1959 Mental Health Act: the experience of ethnic minorities', *New Community*, **13** (1), pp. 86–93.

Ineichen, B., Harrison, G. and Morgan, H. (1984) 'Psychiatric hospital admissions in Bristol', *British Journal of Psychiatry*, **145**, pp. 206–211.

Ingleby, D. (1983) 'Mental health and social order', in Cohen, S. and Scull, A. (Eds) *Social Control and the State*, Oxford, Blackwell.

Ingleby, D. (Ed.) (1981) *Critical Psychiatry*, Harmondsworth, Penguin.

Ismail, K. (1996) 'Planning services for black women', in Abel, K. *et al.* (Eds) *Planning Community Mental Health Services for Women*, London, Routledge.

James, M. and Jongeward, D. (1971) *Born to Win*, Reading, MA, Addison Wesley.

Jay, M. (1973) *The Dialectical Imagination*, London, Heinemann.

Jehu, D. (1990) *Sexual Abuse and Beyond*, Chichester, Wiley.

Jenner, A. (1996/1997) 'Deconstructing over half a century of increasing involvement with psychiatry', *Asylum*, **10** (1), pp. 24–28.

Jenner, A., Monteiro, A. C. D., Zagalo-Cardoso, J. A. and Cunha-Ouveira, J. A. (1993) *Schizophrenia. A Disease or Some Ways of Being Human?*, Sheffield, Sheffield Academic Press.

Jennings, S. (1996) *Creating Solutions. Developing Alternatives in Black Mental Health*, London, King's Fund.

Jodelet, D. (1991) *Madness and Social Representations*, London, Harvester Wheatsheaf.

Johnson, S. and Buszewicz, M. (1996) 'Introduction', in Abel, K. *et al.* (Eds) *Planning Community Mental Health Services for Women*, London, Routledge.

Johnstone, L. (1989) *Users and Abusers of Psychiatry: A Critical Look at Traditional Psychiatric Practice*, London, Routledge.

Jones, G. and Berry, M. (1986) 'Regional secure units: the emerging picture', in Edwards, G. (Ed.) *Current Issues in Clinical Psychology 4*, London, Plenum Press.

Jones, K. (1972) *A History of the Mental Health Services*, London, Routledge and Kegan Paul.

Jones, K. (1993) *Asylums and After*, London, Athlone Press.

Jung, C. G. (1961) *Memories, Dreams, Reflections*, London, Fontana.

Jung, C. G. (1977) *The Psychogenesis of Mental Disease*, London, Routledge and Kegan Paul.

Kane, J. M. and Freeman, H. L. (1994) 'Toward a more effective antipsychotic treatment', *British Journal of Psychiatry*, **165**, Supplement 25, pp. 22–31.

Kaufert, P., Gilbert, P. and Tate, R. (1992) 'The Manitoba Project: a reexamination of the link between menopause and depression', *Maturitas*, **14**, pp. 143–155.

Kelleher, D. and Hillier, S. (Eds) (1996) *Researching Cultural Differences in Health*, London, Routledge.

Kennard, D. (1998) *An Introduction to Therapeutic Communities*, 2nd Edition, London, Jessica Kingsley.

Kennard, D. and Roberts, J. (1983) *An Introduction to Therapeutic Communities*, London, Routledge and Kegan Paul

Kerr, A. (1997) 'Thomas Szasz: in conversation with Alan Kerr', *Psychiatric Bulletin*, **21**, pp. 39–44.

Kingdon, D. and Turkington, D. (1995) *Cognitive-behavioural Therapy of Schizophrenia*, London, Erlbaum.

Kirby, D. (1997) 'The NLP FAQ and Resources', <http://www.rain.org/da5e/nlpfaq.html#What>, accessed July 1998.

Kitzinger, C. and Perkins, R. (1993) *Changing Our Minds: Lesbian Feminism and Psychology*, London, Onlywomen Press.

Knibbs, S. (1994) 'Women on My Mind', *Community Care*, 19–25 May, pp.14–15.

Kohon, G. (Ed.) (1986) *The British School of Psychoanalysis*, London, Free Association Books.

Koss, M. (1990) 'The women's mental health research agenda: violence against women', *American Psychologist*, **45** (3), pp. 374–380.

Kotowicz, Z. (1997) *R. D. Laing and the Paths of Anti-psychiatry*, London, Routledge.

Kuhn, T. (1962) *The Structure of Scientific Revolutions*, Chicago, University of Chicago Press.

Lacey, R. (1983) 'David Cooper: interview by Ron Lacey', *OpenMind*, **3**, pp. 8–9.

Lacey, R. (1995) 'Still pioneering after all these years', in Berke, J. H., Masoliver, C. and Ryan, T. J. (Eds) *Sanctuary*, London, Process Press, pp. 143–152.

Lacey, R. and Woodward, S. (1985) *That's Life! Survey on Tranquillizers*, London, BBC/MIND.

Laing, A. (1994) *R. D. Laing: A Life*, London, HarperCollins.

Laing, R. D. (1959) *The Divided Self*, London, Tavistock.

Laing, R. D. (1965) *The Divided Self*, Harmondsworth, Pelican.

Laing, R. D. (1961) *Self and Others*, Harmondsworth, Penguin.

Laing, R. D. (1967) *The Politics of Experience and the Bird of Paradise*, Harmondsworth, Penguin.

Laing, R. D. (1972) *The Politics of the Family and Other Essays*, London, Tavistock.

Laing, R. D. (1982) *The Voice of Experience*, New York, Pantheon.

Laing, R. D. and Esterson, A. (1964) *Sanity, Madness and the Family*, London, Tavistock.

Lanyon R. I. and Lanyon, B. P. (1978) *What is Behaviour Therapy?*, New York, Addison Wesley.

Latimer, M. (1992) *Funding Black Groups. A Report into Charitable Funding of Ethnic Minority Organisations*, London, Directory of Social Change.

Law, D. (1979) *A Guide to Alternative Medicine*, London, Turnstone.

Laws, S. (1985) *Seeing Red: The Politics of PMT*, London, Hutchinson.

Le Grand, J. and Bartlett, W. (Eds) (1993) *Quasi-markets and Social Policy*, Basingstoke, Macmillan.

Leifer, R. (1990) 'The medical model as the ideology of the therapeutic state', in Cohen, D. (Ed.) *Challenging the Therapeutic State: Critical Perspectives on Psychiatry and the Mental Health System*, Institute of Mind and Behaviour.

Lewis, G., Croft-Jeffreys, C. and David, A. (1990) 'Are British Psychiatrists Racist?', *British Journal of Psychiatry*, **157**, pp. 410–415.

Lewis, J., Bernstock, P. and Bovell, V. (1995) 'The community care changes: unresolved tensions and policy issues in implementation', *Journal of Social Policy*, **24** (1), pp. 73–94.

Lieberman, J. A. and Koreen, A. R. (1993) 'Neurochemistry and neuroendocrinology of schizophrenia: a selective review', *Schizophrenia Bulletin*, **19**, pp. 371–429.

Light, D. (1980) *Becoming Psychiatrists: The Professional Transformation of Self*, Chicago, W. Norton.

Lindow, V. (1990) 'Participation and power', *OpenMind*, **44**, pp. 10–11.

Lindow, V. (1993) 'Survivor, activist or witch', *Asylum*, **7** (4), pp. 5–7.

Littlewood, R. and Cross, S. (1980) 'Ethnic minorities and psychiatric services', *Sociology of Health and Illness*, **2**, pp. 194–201.

Littlewood, R. and Lipsedge, M. (1987) 'The butterfly and the serpent: culture, psychopathology and biomedicine', *Culture, Medicine and Psychiatry*, **11**, pp. 289–335.

Littlewood, R. and Lipsedge, M. (1998) *Aliens and Alienists: Ethnic Minorities and Psychiatry*, 3rd Edition, London, Routledge.

Livingston, G. and Blanchard, M. (1996) 'Planning community mental health services for older women', in Abel, K. *et al.* (Eds) *Planning Community Mental Health Services for Women*, London, Routledge.

Lomax, M. (1921) *The Experiences of an Asylum Doctor*, London, Allen and Unwin.

Loring, M and Powell, B (1988) 'Gender, race and DSM111: a study of the objectivity of psychiatric diagnostic behaviour', *Journal of Health and Social Behaviour*, **29**, pp. 1–22.

Macdonald, M. (1981) *Mystical Bedlam: Madness, Anxiety and Healing in Seventeenth-century England*, Cambridge, Cambridge University Press.

MacFarlane, L. (1998) *Diagnosis: Homophobic. The Experiences of Lesbians, Gay Men and Bisexuals in Mental Health Services*, London, PACE.

Macleod, S. (1981) *The Art of Starvation*, London, Virago.

Marchant, C. (1995) 'Care managers speak out', *Community Care*, 30 March, pp. 16–17.

Martin, J. P. (1984) *Hospitals in Trouble*, Oxford, Blackwell.

Masson, J. (1984) *The Assault on Truth: Freud's Final Abandonment of the Seduction Theory*, London, HarperCollins.

Masson, J. (1990) *Against Therapy*, London, Fontana.

May, T. and Williams, M. (Eds) (1998) *Knowing the Social World*, Buckingham, Open University Press.

McFarland, B. (1991) *Shame and Body Image: Culture and the Compulsive Eater*, Health Communications.

McFarlane, J. M. and Williams, T. M. (1994) 'Placing Premenstrual Syndrome in Perspective', *Psychology of Women Quarterly*, **18**, pp. 339–373.

McGovern, D. and Cope, R. (1987) 'The compulsory detention of males of different ethnic groups with special reference to offender patients', *British Journal of Psychaitry*, **150**, pp. 505–512.

McKinlay, J. B., McKinlay, S. M. and Brambilla, D. J. (1987) 'The relative contributions of endocrine changes and social circumstances to depression in middle-aged women', *Journal of Health and Social Behaviour*, **28**, pp. 345–363.

Mechanic, D. (1969) *Mental Health and Social Policy*, New Jersey, Prentice Hall.

Mental Health Foundation (1994) *Creating Community Care: Report of the Mental Health foundation Inquiry into Community Care for People with Severe Mental Illness*, London, Mental Health Foundation.

Mercer, K. (1986) 'Racism and transcultural psychiatry', in Miller, P. and Rose, N. (Eds) *The Power of Psychiatry*, Cambridge, Polity Press.

Miles, A. (1988) *Women and Mental Illness: The Social Context of Female Neurosis*, Brighton, Wheatsheaf.

Miller, J. (1994) *The Passions of Michel Foucault*, London, Flamingo Press.

Miller, P. (1986) 'Critiques of psychiatry and critical sociologies of madness', in Miller, P. and Rose, N. (Eds) *The Power of Psychiatry*, Cambridge, Polity Press.

Miller, P. and Rose, N. (Eds) (1986) *The Power of Psychiatry*, Cambridge, Polity Press.

Mills, M. (1996) 'Shanti: an intercultural psychotherapy centre for women in the community', in Abel, K. *et al.* (Eds) *Planning Community Mental Health Services for Women*, London, Routledge.

MIND (1993) *MIND's Policy on Black and Minority Ethnic People and Mental Health*, London, MIND.

MIND (1996) 'Risks and rights', *OpenMind*, **80**, April/May, pp. 5–6.

Ministry of Health (1968) *Psychiatric Nursing Today and Tomorrow*, London, HMSO.

Mirowsky, J. and Ross, C. E. (1989) 'Psychiatric diagnosis as reified measurement', *Journal of Health and Social Behaviour*, **30**, pp. 11–25.

Mitchell, J. (1974) *Psychoanalysis and Feminism*, Harmondsworth, Penguin.

Mollica, R. F. and Mills, M. (1986) 'Social class and psychiatric practice: a revision of the Hollingshead and Redlich model', *American Journal of Psychiatry*, **143** (1), pp. 12–17.

Monahan, J. (1992) 'Mental disorder and violent behaviour, perceptions and evidence', *American Psychologist*, **47** (4), pp. 511–521.

Moodley, P. (1995) 'Reaching out', in Fernando, S. (Ed.) *Mental Health in a Multi-ethnic Society: A Multi-disciplinary Handbook*, London, Routledge.

Moodley, P. and Perkins, R. (1991) 'Routes to psychiatric in-patient care in an inner London borough' *Social Psychiatry and Psychiatric Epidemiology*, **26**, pp. 47–51.

Mosher, L. (1996) *The Influence of Research on Health Policy: Walking the Razor's Edge*, Baltimore, University of Maryland School of Social Work (UK source: Planned Environment Therapy Trust Archive, Church Lane, Toddington, Cheltenham GL54 5DQ).

Muijen, M. (1995) 'Mental illness and crime', in *Scare in the Community. Britain in a Moral Panic*, London, Community Care.

Mullan, B. (1995) *Mad to be Normal: Conversations with R.D. Laing*, London, Free Association Books.

National Institute for Social Work (NISW) (1995) *Working in the Social Services*, London, NISW.

Nettleton, S. (1995) *The Sociology of Health and Illness*, London, Polity Press.

Newman, F. (1991) *The Myth of Psychology*, New York, Castillo.

Newman, F. and Holzman, L. (1993a) *Vygotsky: Revolutionary Scientist*, London, Routledge.

Newman, F. and Holzman, L. (1993b) 'Vygotsky, Wittgenstein and Social Therapy', Public Lecture at Manchester Metropolitan University (organized by Psychology, Politics, Resistance), 2 June.

NHS Consultants Association (NHSCA) (1995) *In Practice: The NHS Market*, Banbury, NHSCA/NHS Support Federation.

NHS Health Advisory Service/DHSS/SSI (1988) *Report on Services Provided by Braodmoor Hospital*, London, HMSO.

NHS Management Executive (1994a) *Introduction of Supervision Registers for Mentally Ill People from 1 April 1994 (HSG (94) 5)*, London, Department of Health.

NHS Management Executive (1994b) *Guidance on the Discharge of Mentally Disordered People and their Continuing Care in the Community (HSG (94) 27)*, London, Department of Health.

Nicolson, P. (1986) 'Developing a feminist approach to depression following childbirth', in Wilkinson, S. (Ed.) *Feminist Social Psychology*, Milton Keynes, Open University Press.

Nicolson, P. (1990) 'Understanding post-natal depression: a mother-centred approach', *Journal of Advanced Nursing*, **15**, pp. 689–695.

Nicolson, P. (1991) 'Menstrual cycle research and the construction of female psychology', in Richardson, J. (Ed.) *Cognition and the Menstrual Cycle*, London, Lawrence Erlbaum.

Nicolson, P. (1992) 'Explanations of post-natal depression: structuring knowledge of female psychology', *Research on Language and Social Interaction*, **25**, pp. 75–96.

Nicolson, R. (1998) 'Learning and skill', in Scott, P. and Spencer, C. (Eds) *Psychology: A Contemporary Introduction*, Oxford, Blackwell.

Nolan, P. (1993) *A History of Mental Health Nursing*, London, Chapman and Hall.

Nuffield Provincial Hospitals Trust (1994) *Housing, Homelessness and Health*, London, Nuffield Provincial Hospitals Trust.

Nursing Times Services (1973) *The Psychiatric Nurse as Therapist*, London, Macmillan Journals.

O'Connor, N. and Ryan, J. (1993) *Wild Desires and Mistaken Identities*, London, Virago.

O'Hagan, M. (1993) *Stopovers on My Way Home from Mars: A Winston Churchill Fellowship Report on the Psychiatric Survivor Movement in the USA, Britain and the Netherlands*, London, Survivors Speak Out.

O'Malley, S. and Hall, G. (1990) 'I have no past', in Rolston, B. and Tomlinson, M. (Eds) *Gender, Sexuality and Social Control*, The European Group for the Study of Deviance and Social Control.

O'Sullivan, S. (1982) 'PMT', *Spare Rib*, **116**, March.

Oakley, A. (1976) *Housewife*, Harmondsworth, Penguin.

Oakley, C. (1989) 'Introducing an incomplete project', in Cooper, R. *et al.* (Eds) *Thresholds Between Philosophy and Psychoanalysis: Papers from the Philadelphia Association,* London, Free Association Books.

Offe, C. (1984) *Contradictions of the Welfare State,* London, Hutchinson.

Orbach, S. (1979) *Fat is a Feminist Issue,* London, Hamlyn.

Orbach, S. (1993) *Hunger Strike,* 2nd Edition, Harmondsworth, Penguin.

Outhwaite, W. (1987) *New Philosophies of Social Science: Realism, Hermeneutics and Critical Theory,* London, Macmillan.

Owusu-Bempah, J. (1989) 'The new institutional racism', *Community Care,* **780,** pp. 23–25.

Parker, I. (1995) '"Right", said Fred, "I'm too sexy for bourgeois group therapy": the case of the Institute for Social Therapy', *Changes,* **13** (1), pp. 1–22.

Parker, I., Georgaca, E., Harper, D., Mclaughlin, T. and Stowell-Smith, M. (1995) *Deconstructing Psychopathology,* London, Sage.

Parry-Jones, W. (1972) *The Trade in Lunacy,* London, Routledge and Kegan Paul.

Parsons, T. (1951) *The Social System,* New York, Free Press.

Parton, N. (1991) *Governing the Family: Child Care, Child Protection and the State,* London, Macmillan.

Pattison, S. (1997) *The Faith of the Managers,* London, Cassell.

Payne, S., (1991) *Women, Health and Poverty – An Introduction,* Hemel Hempstead, Harvester Wheatsheaf.

Pedler, M. and Foster, S. (1998) 'Laying down the law?', *OpenMind,* **94,** pp. 6–7.

Pembroke, L. (1994) *Self-harm: Perspectives from Personal Experience,* London, Survivors Speak Out.

Pembroke, L., Smith, A. and National Self-Harm Network (1996) *Self Injury – Myths and Common Sense* (A double-sided A4 information sheet available through Survivors Speak Out, 34 Osnaburgh Street, London NW1).

Penfold, P. S. and Walker, G. A. (1984) *Women and the Psychiatric Paradox,* Milton Keynes, Open University Press.

Perceval, J. (1838/40) *A Narrative of the Treatment Received/Experienced by a Gentleman During a State of Mental Derangement,* London, Effingham Wilson.

Perkins, R. (1999a) 'Joined-up government?', *OpenMind,* **96,** p. 6.

Perkins, R. (1999b) 'ECT: a dissenting view', *OpenMind,* **97,** p. 15.

Perkins, R. E. (1996) 'Women, lesbians and community care', in Abel, K. *et al.* (Eds) *Planning Community Mental Health Services for Women,* London, Routledge.

Persaud, R. (1995) on BBC2, *States of Mind: The Talking Cure,* London, BBC Television, 2 February.

Peterson, D. (1977) *The Literature of Madness: Autobiographical Writings by Mad People and Mental Patients in England and America from 1436–1975,* unpublished PhD Dissertation, Stanford University.

Philo, G. (1996) *Media and Mental Distress,* Glasgow Media Group, Longman.

Philo, G., Secker, J., Platt, S., Henderson, L., McLaughlin, G. and Bornside,

J. (1994) 'The impact of the mass media on public opinion of mental illness', *Health Education Journals*, **53**, pp. 271–281.

Pilgrim, D. (1992a) 'Competing histories of madness', in Bentall, R. P. (Ed.) *Reconstructing Schizophrenia*, London, Routledge.

Pilgrim, D. (1992b) 'Rhetoric and nihilism in mental health policy', *Critical Social Policy*, **34**, pp. 106–113.

Pilgrim, D. (1993) 'Mental Health Services in the Twenty-first Century: The User-Professional Divide?', in Bornat, J. *et al.* (Eds) *Community Care: A Reader*, London, Macmillan/Open University Press.

Pilgrim, D. (1997) *Psychotherapy and Society*, London, Sage.

Pilgrim, D. (1999) 'Badly in need of help', *OpenMind*, **95**, p. 7.

Pilgrim, D. and Rogers, A. (1993) *A Sociology of Mental Health and Illness*, Buckingham, Open University Press.

Pilgrim, D. and Rogers, A. (1998) 'Six points in search of policy', *OpenMind*, **89**, pp. 10–11.

Pilgrim, D. and Treacher, A. (1992) *Clinical Psychology Observed*, London, Routledge.

Pinto, R. (1970) 'A study of Asians in the Camberwell area', unpublished MPhil Dissertation, University of London.

Pipe, R., Bhat, A., Mathews, B. and Hampstead, J. (1991) 'Section 136 and African/Afro-Caribbean minorities', *International Journal of Social Psychiatry*, **37** (1), pp. 14–23.

Porter, R. (1987a) *Mind-forg'd Manacles*, London, Athlone.

Porter, R. (1987b) *A Social History of Madness: Stories of the Insane*, London, Weidenfeld and Nicolson.

Prins, H. (1980) *Offenders, Deviants or Patients? An Introduction to the Study of Socio-forensic Problems*, London, Tavistock.

Prins, H., Blacker-Holst, T., Francis, E. and Keitch, I. (1993) *Report of the Committee of Inquiry into the Death in Broadmoor Hospital of Orville Blackwood and a Review of the Deaths of Two Other Afro-Caribbean Patients. Big, Black and Dangerous?*, London, SHSA.

Prior, C. (1998) 'Future imperfect?', *Community Care*, 26 February–4 March, pp. 22–23.

Prior, L. (1991) 'Mind, body and behaviour: theorisations of madness and the organisation of therapy', *Sociology*, **25** (3), pp. 403–422.

Prior, L. (1993) *The Social Organization of Mental Illness*, London, Sage.

Rachman, S. (1971) *The Effects of Psychotherapy*, Oxford, Pergamon Press.

Rack, P. (1982) *Race, Culture and Mental Disorder*, London, Tavistock.

Radical Therapist Collective (1974) *The Radical Therapist*, Harmondsworth, Pelican.

Ramon, S. (1985) *Psychiatry in Britain: Meaning and Policy*, London, Croom Helm.

Ramon, S. (1996) *Mental Health in Europe: Ends, Beginnings and Rediscoveries*, London, Macmillan.

Redding, K. (1996) *Transsexual Syndrome*, London, Trinity Workshop/Change.

Reich, W. (1970) *The Mass Psychology of Fascism*, London, Souvenir Press.

Reich, W. (1975a) *Reich Speaks of Freud*, Harmondsworth, Pelican.

Reich, W. (1975b) *Listen, Little Man!*, Harmondsworth, Pelican.

Reinharz, S. (1993) 'The principles of feminist research: a matter of debate', in Kramarae, C. and Spender, D. (Eds) *The Knowledge Explosion: Generations of Feminist Scholarship*, Hemel Hempstead, Harvester Wheatsheaf.

Rich, A. (1976) *Of Woman Born: Motherhood as Experience and Institution*, New York, Norton.

Ridley, M. (1993) *The Red Queen*, London, Viking.

Rieker, P. P. and Jankowski, M. K. (1995) 'Sexism and women's psychological status', in Willie, C. V. *et al.* (Eds) *Mental Health, Racism and Sexism*, London, Taylor & Francis.

Ritchie, J. H., Dick, D. and Lingham, R. (1994) *The Report of the Inquiry into the Care and Treatment of Christopher Clunis*, London, HMSO.

Roberts, H. (1985) *The Patient Patients*, London, Pandora.

Roberts, M. (1997) 'Survivor outrage and genetic research into so-called mental disorders', *Survivors Speak Out Newssheet*, May, pp. 10–11.

Roberts, R. (1990) 'Psychiatry, science and mental health: arguments against medical tyranny', *Critical Public Health*, **4**, pp. 15–20.

Rogers, A, Pilgrim, D. and Lacey, R. (1993) *Experiencing Psychiatry: Users' Views of Services*, London, Macmillan.

Rogers, A. and Faulkner, A. (1987) *A Place of Safety*, London, MIND.

Rogers, A. and Pilgrim, D. (1991) 'Pulling down the churches: accounting for the British Mental Health Users' Movement', *Sociology of Health and Illness*, **13** (2), pp. 129–147.

Rogers, A. and Pilgrim, D. (1996) *Mental Health Policy in Britain: A Critical Introduction*, Houndmills, Macmillan.

Rogers, C. (1951) *Client-centred Therapy*, London, Constable.

Rogers, C. (1980) *A Way of Being*, Boston, Houghton Mifflin.

Romme, M. and Escher, S. (1993) *Accepting Voices*, London, Macmillan.

Romme, M. and Escher, S. (1996) 'Empowering people who hear voices', in Haddock, G. and Slade, P. D. (Eds) *Cognitive-behavioural Interventions with Psychotic Disorders*, London, Routledge.

Rooney, B. (1987) *Racism and Resistance to Change*, Liverpool, Merseyside Area Profile Group.

Rose, N. (1979) 'The psychological complex: mental measurement and social administration', *Ideology and Consciousness*, **5**, Spring, pp. 5–68.

Rose, N. (1985) *The Psychology Complex: Psychology, Politics and Society in England 1869–1939*, London, Routledge and Kegan Paul.

Rose, N. (1986) 'Law, rights and psychiatry', in Miller, P. and Rose, N. (Eds) *The Power of Psychiatry*, Cambridge, Cambridge University Press.

Rose, N. (1989) 'Individualizing psychology', in Shotter, J. and Gergen, K. J. (Eds) *Texts of Identity*, London, Sage.

Rose, N. (1990) *Governing the Soul*, London, Routledge.

Rose, N. (1992) *Romme and Escher: The Dutch Experience*, Manchester, Hearing Voices Network.

Rothman, D. (1971) *The Discovery of the Asylum: Social Order and Disorder in the New Republic*, Boston, Little Brown.

Rowley, H. and Grosz, E. (1992) 'Psychoanalysis and feminism', in Gunew, S. (Ed.) *Feminist Knowledge: Critique and Construct*, London, Routledge.

Rushton, J. P. (1988) 'Race differences in behaviour: a review and evolutionary analysis', *Personality and Individual Difference*, **9** (6), pp. 1009–1024.

Rushton, J. P. (1990) 'Race differences, r/k theory and a reply to Flynn', *The Psychologist*, **5**, pp. 195–198.

Russell, D. (1995) *Women, Madness and Medicine*, Cambridge, Polity Press.

Russell, D. (1997) *Scenes from Bedlam: A History of Caring for the Mentally Disordered at Bethlem Royal Hospital and the Maudsley*, London, Bailliere Tindall.

Rutter, P. (1995) *Sex in the Forbidden Zone: When Men in Power Abuse Women's Trust*, London, Aquarian.

Rwgellera, G. G. C. (1977) 'Psychiatric morbidity among West Africans and West Indians living in London', *Psychological Medicine*, **7**, pp. 317–329.

Salkovskis, P. (1993) 'Editorial', *Behavioural and Cognitive Psychotherapy*, **21** (2), p. 169.

Sapsford, R. J. (1981) 'Individual deviance: the search for the criminal personality', in Fitzgerald, M. *et al.* (Eds) *Crime and Society*, London, Routledge/Open University Press.

Sashidharan, S. P. (1986) 'Ideology and politics in transcultural psychiatry', in Cox, J. L. (Ed.) *Transcultural Psychiatry*, London, Croom Helm.

Sashidharan, S. P. (1994) 'Opposing and resisting: a view from the Third World', *Asylum*, **8** (1), pp. 31–34.

Schatzman, M. (*circa* 1980) *The Story of Ruth*, New York, Zebra Books. No date of publication is given in this edition, but the hardback edition was published in 1980 by G. P. Putnam.

Scheff, T. (1966) *Being Mentally Ill: A Sociological Theory*, Chicago, Aldine.

Scheper-Hughes, N. and Lovell, A. M. (1987) *Psychiatry Inside Out: Selected Writings of Franco Basaglia*, New York, Columbia University Press.

Schizophrenia Media Agency (1995) *Schizophrenia Media Agency*, Pamphlet, Manchester, SMA.

Schooler, N. (1991) 'Maintenance medication for schizophrenia: strategies for dose reduction', *Schizophrenia Bulletin*, **17**, pp. 311–324.

Scull, A. (1977) *Decarceration. Community Treatment and the Deviant. A Radical View*, New Jersey, Prentice Hall.

Scull, A. (1979) *Museums of Madness: the Social Organization of Insanity in Nineteenth Century England*, London, Allen Lane.

Scull, A. (1981) *Mad Houses, Mad Doctors and Madmen: the Social History of Psychiatry in the Victorian Era*, London, Athlone.

Scull, A. (1989) *Social Order/Mental Disorder: Anglo-American Psychiatry in Historical Perspective*, London, Routledge.

Scull, A. (1993) *The Most Solitary of Afflictions: Madness and Society in Britain, 1700–1900*, New Haven, Yale University Press.

Sedgwick, P. (1982) *Psychopolitics*, London, Pluto Press.

'Seeger, Pete' (1996) 'A concise political history of the user movement', *Asylum*, **9** (4), pp. 12–13.

Seldon, A. (Ed.) (1985) *The New Right Enlightenment*, Sevenoaks, Economic and Literary Books.

Shaikh, S. (1985) 'Cross-cultural comparison: psychiatric admissions of Asian and indigenous patients in Leicestershire', *International Journal of Social Psychiatry*, **31**, pp. 3–11.

Sharpe, S. (1984) *Double Identity: The Lives of Working Mothers*, Harmondsworth, Penguin.

Sheppard, D. (1995) *Learning the Lessons: Mental Health Inquiry Reports Published in England and Wales Between 1969–1994 and their Recommendations for Improving Practice*, London, Institute of Mental Health Law/The Zito Trust.

Sheppard, M. (1991) 'General practice, social work and mental health sections: the social control of women', *British Journal of Social Work*, **21**, pp. 663–683.

Showalter, E. (1987) *The Female Malady: Women, Madness and English Culture, 1830–1980*, London, Virago.

Sigal, C. (1986) 'The doctor who opened the door to the people at Villa 21', *The Guardian*, 27 August, p. 11.

Sim, M. (1981) *Guide to Psychiatry*, Edinburgh, Churchill Livingstone.

Skinner, B. F. (1973) *Beyond Freedom and Dignity*, Harmondsworth, Pelican.

Skinner, B. F. (1974) *About Behaviourism*, London, Jonathan Cape.

Skultans, V. (1975) *Madness and Morals: Ideas on Insanity in the Nineteenth Century*, London, Routledge and Kegan Paul.

Sluka, J. A. (1989) 'Living on their nerves: nervous debility in Northern Ireland', in Davis, D. L. and Low, S. M. (Eds) *Gender, Health and Illness: The Case of Nerves*, New York, Hemisphere.

Smith, A. (1998) 'Use it or lose it', *OpenMind*, **91**, pp. 10–11..

Spandler, H. (1992) 'To make an army out of an illness', *Asylum*, **6** (4), pp. 4–16.

Stancombe, J. and White, S. (1998) 'Psychotherapy without foundations? Hermeneutics, discourse and the end of certainty, *Theory and Psychology*, **8** (5), pp. 579–599.

Stanton, H. E. (1996) 'Combining hypnosis and NLP in the treatment of telephone phobia', *Australian Journal of Clinical and Experimental Hypnosis*, **24** (1), pp. 53–58.

Steele, L. (1998) 'Mind games', *Community Care*, 3–9 December.

Stevens, J. O. (1975) *Gestalt Is*, Moab, UT, Real People Press.

Stewart, I. and Joines, V. (1987) *TA Today*, Nottingham, Lifespace.

Stone, M. (1985) 'Shell-shock and the psychologists', in Bynum, W. F. *et al.* (Eds) *The Anatomy of Madness: Essays in the History of Psychiatry*, Volume 2, London, Tavistock.

Stoppard, J. M. (1997) 'Women's bodies, women's lives and depression: towards a reconciliation of material and discursive accounts', in Ussher, J. M. (Ed.) *Body Talk: The Material and Discursive Regulation of Sexuality, Madness and Reproduction*, London, Routledge.

Subotsky, F. (1996) 'Girls in distress: an unconsidered issue', in Abel, K. *et al.* (Eds) *Planning Community Mental Health Services for Women*, London, Routledge.

Surrey, J, Swett, C., Michaels, B. and Levin, S. (1990) 'Reported history of physical and sexual abuse and severity of symptomatology in women psychiatric outpatients', *American Orthopsychiatrist*, **60** (3), pp. 412–417.

Survivors Speak Out (1986) *We're Not Mad, We're Angry*, London, Multiple Image.

Survivors Speak Out (1997) 'Reclaim Bedlam Campaign', *Survivors Speak Out Newssheet*, May, p. 5.

Swann, C. (1997) 'Reading the bleeding body: discourses of premenstrual syndrome', in Ussher, J. M. (Ed.) *Body Talk: The Material and Discursive Regulation of Sexuality, Madness and Reproduction*, London, Routledge.

Szasz, T. S. (1961) *The Myth of Mental Illness*, New York, Hoeber-Harper.

Szasz, T. S. (1963) *Law, Liberty and Psychiatry*, New York, Macmillan.

Szasz, T.S. (1971) *The Manufacture of Madness*, London, Routledge and Kegan Paul.

Szasz, T. S. (1978) 'Pilgrim's regress', *The Spectator*, **241**, No. 7838 pp. 72–73.

Szasz, T. S. (1979a) *The Myth of Psychotherapy*, Oxford, Oxford University Press.

Szasz, T. S. (1979b) *Schizophrenia: The Sacred Symbol of Psychiatry*, Oxford, Oxford University Press.

Szasz, T. S. (1990) 'Law and psychiatry: the problems that will not go away', in Cohen, D. (Ed.) *Challenging the Therapeutic State: Critical Perspectives on Psychiatry and the Mental Health System*, Institute of Mind and Behaviour.

Szasz, T. S. (1994) *Cruel Compassion*, Chichester, Wiley and Sons.

Tame, C. (1991) 'Freedom, responsibility and justice: the criminology of the 'new right', in Stenson, K. and Cowell, D. (Eds) *The Politics of Crime Control*, London, Sage.

Taylor, D. (1987) 'Current usage of benzodiazepines in Britain', in Freeman, H. and Rue, Y. (Eds) *Benzodiazepines in Current Clinical Practice*, London, Royal Society of Medicine Services.

Taylor, P. J. and Gunn, J. (1999) 'Homicides by people with mental illness: myth and reality', *British Journal of Psychiatry*, **174**, pp. 9–14.

Taylor, R. (1994/95) 'Alienation and integration in mental health policy', *Critical Social Policy*, **42**, Winter.

Thomas, A. and Sillen, S. (1972) *Racism and Psychiatry*, New York, Brunner/Mazel.

Thomas, C. S., Stone, K., Osborn, M., Thomas, P. F. and Fisher, M. (1993) 'Psychiatric morbidity and compulsory admission among UK-born Europeans, Afro-Caribbeans and Asians in Central Manchester', *British Journal of Psychiatry*, **163**, pp. 91–99.

Thomas, P. (1997) *The Dialectics of Schizophrenia*, London, Free Association Books.

Thomas, P. and Bracken, P. (1999) 'Putting patients first', *OpenMind*, **96**, pp. 14–15.

Thompson, N. (1993) *Anti-discriminatory Practice*, London, Macmillan.

Ticktin, S. (1997) Telephone conversation with John Hopton, 31 January.

Tomes, N. (1988) 'The great restraint controversy: a comparative perspective on Anglo-American psychiatry in the nineteenth century', in Bynum, W. F. *et al.* (Eds) *The Anatomy of Madness: Essays in the History of Madness*, Volume 3, London, Routledge.

Torkington, P. (1983) *The Racial Politics of Health: A Liverpool Profile*, Liverpool, Merseyside Area Profile Group.

Torkington, P. (1991) *Black Health – A Political Issue*, London, Catholic Association for Racial Justice.

Treacher, A. and Baruch, G. (1981) 'Towards a critical history of the psychiatric profession', in Ingleby, D. (Ed.) *Critical Psychiatry: The Politics of Mental Health*, Harmondsworth, Penguin.

Trower, P., Casey, A. and Dryden, W. (1988) *Cognitive-behavioural Counselling in Action*, London, Sage.

Turner, T. (1988) 'Henry Maudsley: psychiatrist, philosopher, and entrepreneur', in Bynum, W. F. *et al.* (Eds) *The Anatomy of Madness: Essays in the History of Madness*, Volume 3, London, Routledge.

Ussher, J. M. (1989) *The Psychology of the Female Body*, London, Routledge.

Ussher, J. M. (1991) *Women's Madness: Misogyny or Mental Illness?*, Hemel Hempstead, Harvester Wheatsheaf.

Ussher, J. M. (1992) 'Science sexing psychology', in Ussher, J. M. and Nicolson, P. (Eds) *Gender Issues in Clinical Psychology*, London, Routledge.

Ussher, J. M. (1997) *Body Talk: The Material and Discursive Regulation of Sexuality, Madness and Reproduction*, London, Routledge.

Valentine, R. (1996) *Asylum, Hospital, Haven – a History of Horton Hospital*, London, Riverside Mental Health Trust.

Van Dusen, W. (1975) 'The Phenomenology of Schizophrenic Existence', in Stevens, J. O. (Eds) *Gestalt Is*, Moab, UT, Real People Press.

Victor, C. R. (1991) *Health and Health Care in Later Life*, Buckingham, Open University Press.

Virden , P. (1996) 'The wing of madness – the life and work of R.D. Laing by David Burston', *Asylum*, **9** (4), pp. 44–50.

Von Bergen, C. W., Soper, B., Rosenthal, G. T. and Wilkinson, L. V. (1997) 'Selected alternative training techniques in HRD', *Human Resource Development Quarterly*, **8** (4), pp. 281–294.

Walker, A. (1995) 'Theory and methodology in premenstrual syndrome research', *Social Science and Medicine*, **41** (6), pp. 793–800.

Wallcraft, J. (1996) 'Some models of asylum and help in times of crisis', in Tomlinson, D. and Carrier, J. (Eds) *Asylum in the Community*, London, Routledge.

Walton, A. (1996/1997) 'Guilty without trial', *Asylum*, **10** (1), p. 35.

Waters, M. (1994) *Modern Sociological Theory*, London, Sage.

Watkins, J. (1996) *Living with Schizophrenia*, Melbourne, Hill of Content.

Watson, G. and Williams, J. (1992) 'Feminist therapy in practice', in Ussher, J. M. and Nicolson, P. (Eds) *Gender Issues in Clinical Psychology*, London, Routledge.

Webb-Johnson, A. (1991) *A Cry for Change. An Asian Perspective on Developing Quality Mental Health Care*, London, Confederation of Indian Organisations.

Weinberg, T. S. (1995) *S & M: Studies in Dominance and Submission*, Amherst, NY, Prometheus.

Weissman, M. and Klerman, G. (1977) 'Sex differences and the epidemiology of depression', *Archives of General Psychiatry*, **34**, pp. 98–111.

Weldon, F. (1994) 'Will no-one rid us of these turbulent priests?', *The Times*, Supplement, 4 February, pp. 8–14.

Wenham, M. (1993) *Funded to Fail – Nuff Pain No Gain*, London, London Voluntary Service Council.

Williams, J. (1993) 'What is a profession? Experience versus expertise', in Walmsley, J. *et al.* (Eds) *Health, Welfare and Practice: Reflecting on Roles and Relationships*, London, Sage/Open University Press.

Wilson, E. (1977) *Women and the Welfare State*, London, Tavistock.

Wilson, M. (1993) *Mental Health and Britain's Black Communities*, London, King's Fund.

Wing, J. K. (1978) *Reasoning about Madness*, Oxford, Oxford University Press.

Wing, J. K. and Freudenberg, R. K. (1961) 'The response of severely ill chronic schizophrenic patients to social stimulation', *American Journal of Psychiatry*, **118**, p. 311.

Wolf, N. (1990) *The Beauty Myth*, London, Chatto and Windus.

Wolpe, J. (1973) *The Practice of Behavior Therapy*, New York, Pergamon.

Wood, D. (1993) *The Power of Words. Uses and Abuses of Talking Treatments*, London, MIND.

World Health Organization (1992) *The ICD-10 Classification of Mental and Behavioural Disorders*, Geneva, WHO.

Wyatt, R. J. (1991) 'Neuroleptics and the natural course of schizophrenia', *Schizophrenia Bulletin*, **17**(2) pp. 325–351.

Zikis, P. (1983) 'Treatment of an 11 year old obsessive-compulsive ritualizer and Tiqueur girl with *in vivo* exposure and response prevention', *Behavioural Psychotherapy*, **11** (1), pp. 75–81.

Zola, I. (1972) 'Medicine as an institution of social control', *Sociological Review*, **20**, pp. 487–503.

Index